Live Consciously, Catch Health

The 8 Pillars to Health & Wholeness

Rita Hari

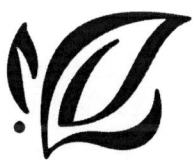

To contact the author, visit www.ritahariwellness.com

KAKCO Publishing
P. O. Box 20664
Columbus, OH 43220

© Rita Hari, 2017

Published 1 January, 2017

Publisher: KAKCO Publishing

Cover design by Amy Magella Gigena

Developmental editing by Sarah Barbour

ISBN-13: 978-0692824962
ISBN-10: 0692824960

Printed in the United States of America

Table of Contents

To the lady who taught me by example how to move through anything with grace and dignity ... my beautiful Mom. I also dedicate this book to anyone who has felt stuck, scared or broken. I sit with you. I stand with you. I walk forward with you.

The seed of this book was planted years ago, but only because of the encouragement, support, and love of many has it taken life.

♡ To Willis, who never really knows exactly what I'm up to but unconditionally supports me: thank you for never clipping my wings.

♡ Thanks to my children, who teach me every day the art of presence and for reminding me that I can be anything when I grow up.

♡ To my sisters, thank you for being by my side. Gita, our daily morning calls lift my days and make things better.

♡ Lindsey, Sue and Joshua from IIN. Thank you for your guidance and for blazing the trail so I could discover my path.

♡ Sarah B., your belief in this book and in my message truly gave it legs … I thank you.

♡ To Amy G., I felt your light shine my way every step of the way on this book journey. You helped me carry the baton to the finish line. I am forever grateful … thank you, my unexpected friend.

♡ Lastly, I am grateful to the beautiful souls who show up to my yoga classes every day. Your honest practice on the mat encourages me to live mine off the mat. The light within me acknowledges the light within you. Thank you. xoxo

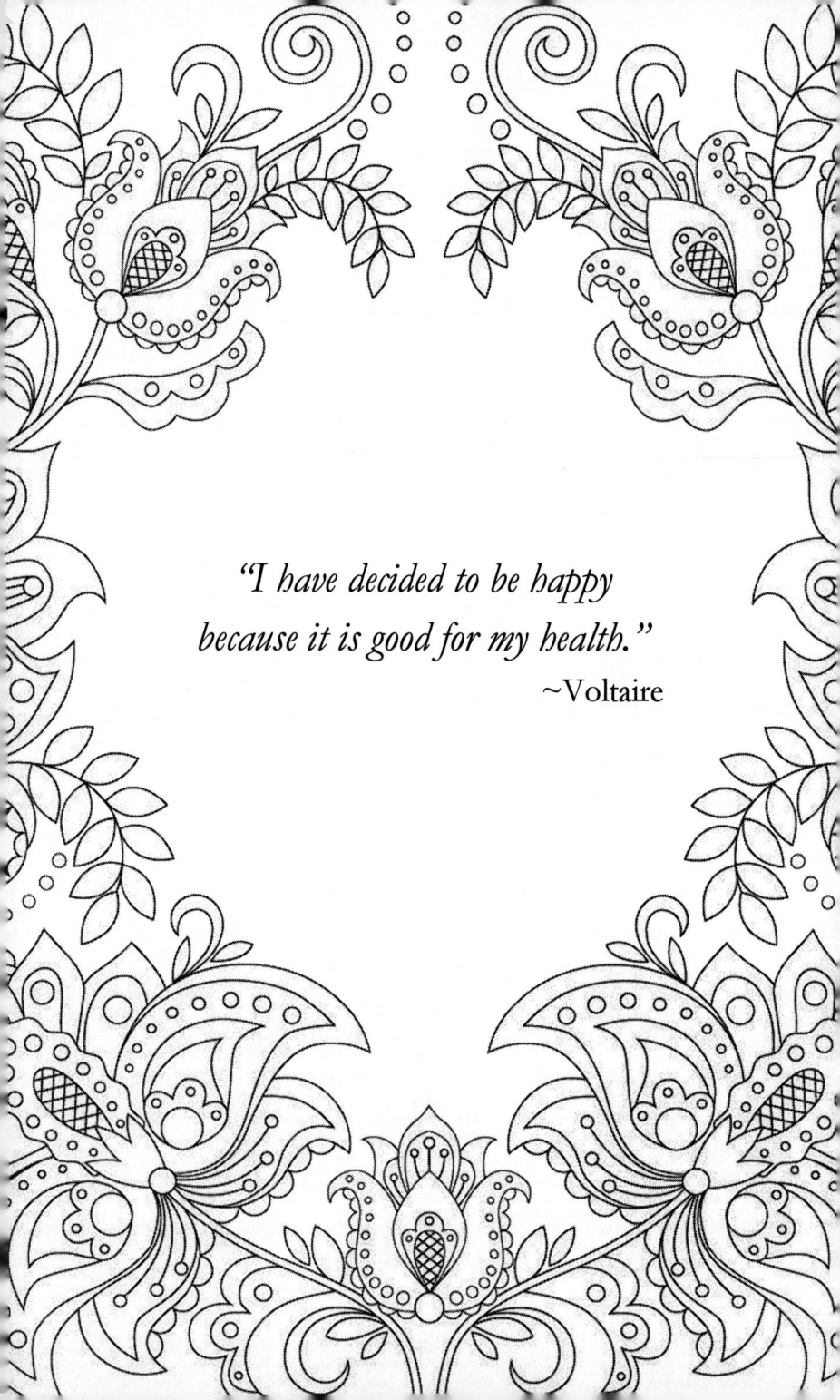

"I have decided to be happy
because it is good for my health."

~Voltaire

Introduction

I don't really believe in accidents.

Throughout the time I was writing this book, I pictured the exact person who would be drawn to it. This book is for someone who wants to experience true wellness and vibrant energy in their body and in their life. A person who is tired of conventional dieting, feeling bad about themselves, and not getting lasting results. Maybe there was a demarcation point in your life—a loss or an unexpected diagnosis; or maybe you've always been a caregiver, and the sheer busyness of your life has taken you away from taking care of yourself. The person I imagine holding this book is someone who feels frustrated and sometimes overwhelmed with their health and the direction life is taking them, yet is also hopeful, and deep inside knows there is more.

If this describes you, this book will set you on your path. It doesn't matter where you are on your health journey; the Eight Pillars of Lasting Health & Wholeness discussed in this book will gently guide you to your destination and beyond. I say "beyond" because I believe getting healthy is just the beginning. Once you start feeling better, you'll start thinking more clearly, and the possibilities of what you can do and be open up.

Who knows what's possible?

What I do know is that you've taken the first step.

So CONGRATULATIONS to both of us … we found each other! Here's to our journey together. High five and big, warm hug. You have landed.

My deepest desire for this book is that it will remind you of your own power to get healthy and happy.

Yes, I said *remind.* You, my friend, already know this, but most of us have forgotten. Do me a favor: from today on, every time you read, hear or see something that touches you in some way—maybe your heart space softens or the depths of your belly pulses—stop, pause and feel it. Maybe it's a line from a poem or a song, a book, a quote, or being in nature … Whatever lights you up, do yourself a favor and remember to stop, pause and feel it. Take it in and capture whatever it is. That, my dear, is your essence, your intuition, your inner-knowing, and it is your most valuable compass. It will lead you to a truer you, and a truer you will lead you to a healthier, happier you. I promise.

This book stems from a deeply rooted belief that when we live consciously, we stop chasing health and false happiness. When we live mindfully, health and inner joy come *to* us. All we have to do is catch them. My intention is for you to not simply learn my Eight Pillars intellectually, but to experience them. It's important for you to find the things that speak to you along the way and make them your own. This is your personalized health journey.

Oh, and please, *take action.* It's important to take action, because knowing without doing is useless. Don't get caught up in the "Yeah, yeah, I know that already" or "That's not new" mindset.

I'm going to let you in on something: *none* of it's new, and it's the small stuff done consistently that pulls us to the next level of health and happiness. What happens over time is that the small, consistent steps we take to better our health become our anchors. Throughout the book, I will suggest some anchors for you to focus on. Pick the ones that speak to you and implement them right away. With your anchors in place, you will be rooted and you will run out of excuses for getting sidetracked. Any number of things, from socializing to traveling to serious life challenges, can throw us off track, but with your anchors in place to support you, you will feel pulled back onto your path. Pulled back gently, never pushed.

Sound good? All right, let's get into it. Again, thank you for picking up this book. I am honored and privileged to be on this journey with you. My heart and support is with you every step of the way.

How to Get the Most Out of This Book

- Get yourself a journal and maybe even a buddy. Accountability is key, and having someone with you will keep you on track—plus it's more fun.

- Stay open and curious to the ideas and suggestions. Remember, it might not be new to you, but *you* taking action brings in the newness. Implement the ideas that speak to you and be consistent.

- In each chapter, I have a series of "Ask Yourself ..." questions. Some questions are designed to get you thinking about what's going on in your own life, where you might be getting stuck or sabotaging yourself. Others are meant for you to take action on and implement. This is an invitation for you to reflect back to your own life, so when you see "Ask Yourself ..." stop reading and take the time to journal your response—and feel free to jot down any other notes or ideas that come up for you along the way.

- Implement one to three recommendations for a couple of weeks and see how you do.

- Once you feel comfortable, toss in a couple more. Make them a habit and a part of your life. This process is not linear, and there is no perfect offering. Our job is to decide what we want, set some goals, and take action again and again. Each day we show up and start where we are.

- Sign-up for my private Facebook group, Catch Health (www.ritahariwellness.com/Facebook). Just send me a request and I will add you in. Our members support each other and hold each other accountable.

- Lastly, trust in the process. Be patient with yourself, and please, know that you deserve health and happiness.

Would you believe me if I told you how magnificent you are, and that *you matter*? I'm writing this book because I believe that somewhere along the way, most of us have forgotten this truth. An event, a person or people, or a situation pushed us away from our natural state, and we dimmed our light.

I call this a broken moment, and a broken moment can lead to a broken state. For some, it may be abrupt—a single, defining moment. For others, it might be a chipping away of their self-worth that takes place over decades. It doesn't matter. If you are not feeling grace and love, you have been robbed. Something or someone, without your consent, hijacked your joy like a thief in the night, and at some point, fear, doubt and worry stepped in and started running your life.

I'm going to get this out right out of the gate: our natural state is love in all its forms—joy, laughter, compassion, abundance, wisdom, creativity and beauty. Everything else has been falsely created. Our true nature is love.

So why is it so hard?

What and how you eat is vital for great health, but honestly, you probably already know what to eat (and what not to). And even if I gave you a list of approved foods and drinks (which I will) and told you to make sure you do some form of exercise an hour a day, would that be enough? No, I don't think it would. Health, Diet and Nutrition is a $70 billion (yes, with a B) industry, yet we are fatter, sicker and more stressed than ever before. Our children, for the first time, are on track to have a shorter life expectancy than their parents. One in every three Americans is considered overweight or obese. This is not okay.

I once heard Tony Robbins say, "If something is not working, ask a better question."

Here is my attempt to ask better questions:

Why do we keep doing what we do, even though we know what we know?

Why is it so hard to make the lasting changes needed to get healthy and feel great?

My answer is simple: we have forgotten our innate power and we have lost the ability to truly love ourselves. I believe that once you get a glimpse of your awesomeness and start caring for yourself, not just by getting a pedicure or massage (don't get me wrong—I heart both) but by treating yourself with kindness, you will naturally do the things that bring you health and happiness. It won't be a diet or a sacrifice; it will be a choice. It will be a lifestyle. The starting point is *your thoughts*. Become your own best friend in your head and the world is yours. Cultivate a loving relationship toward yourself and your world will change. This is my promise.

These Eight Pillars to Health & Wholeness will build a foundation for a healthier, happier, more fulfilling life:

1. Your Inner Circle

2. Water

3. Sleep

4. Movement

5. Stress Management

6. Connection to Something Bigger

7. Pockets of Joy

8. Food

I will break down each of the Eight Pillars and give you all the secrets and tips you need to know to start right away. I don't want you to make the same mistakes I did during my healing process; I got stuck in quicksand and did not have the tools to help myself. Not you, though—you will have the tools. While the Pillars are all equally important, some may be more important *for you* at this stage in your life. By the end of this book, you will recognize what areas of your life need more attention, in order to feel your best. Pick an area you know needs some attention and start there.

One more thing before we start our journey together: throughout this book, I invite you to stop, take a moment, and just *breathe*. Even though it's something we do all day, every day, the entire length of our lives, most of us never take a moment to consciously focus on our breath. Whether you take a single conscious breath or meditate for an hour, Buddha belly breaths are an easy way to develop a mindful breathing practice.

Buddha belly breaths:

- Sit on the floor or on a chair in an easy cross-legged position. Sit nice and tall.

- Close your eyes.

- Gently drop your shoulders.

- Check in with the body.

- Notice your breath. Notice the length, the quality and the texture.

- Are the inhales and exhales the same length?

- Breathe in and out the nose and settle into the breath. Begin to smooth it out and allow the breath to soothe you.

- With every inhale, feel as though you are receiving prana (life force).

- With every exhale is a letting go.

- Soften your throat, the back of your eyes and your belly.

- Put your hands on your lower belly.

- With every inhale feel the belly expand and fill.

- With every exhale, the naval draws in toward the spine and the belly contracts.

- Find a rhythm that you are comfortable with and take ten deep Buddha belly breaths.

- After ten breaths, you can release your hands onto your legs, keep your eyes closed and notice how you feel. No judgment, just observation.

Right now, take several deep Buddha belly breaths and allow your body to relax. Seriously, do it—this is one of those small things you might overlook. Allow the breath to flood the mind and let go of all the thoughts that are not serving you at this moment. Let go of what you think you know. Let go of what you think you can't do and allow the breath to lead. I am with you every step of the way.

Ask Yourself ...

- What would it be like if you had love and acceptance for your body?

- How would you be different in the world?

- How would you walk?

- How would you dress?

- What goals would you set and achieve?

- How would you show up in the world?

Trust in the process and get ready to once and for all take back your health, reclaim your innate power, and activate your true nature—which happens to be *healthy* and *happy.*

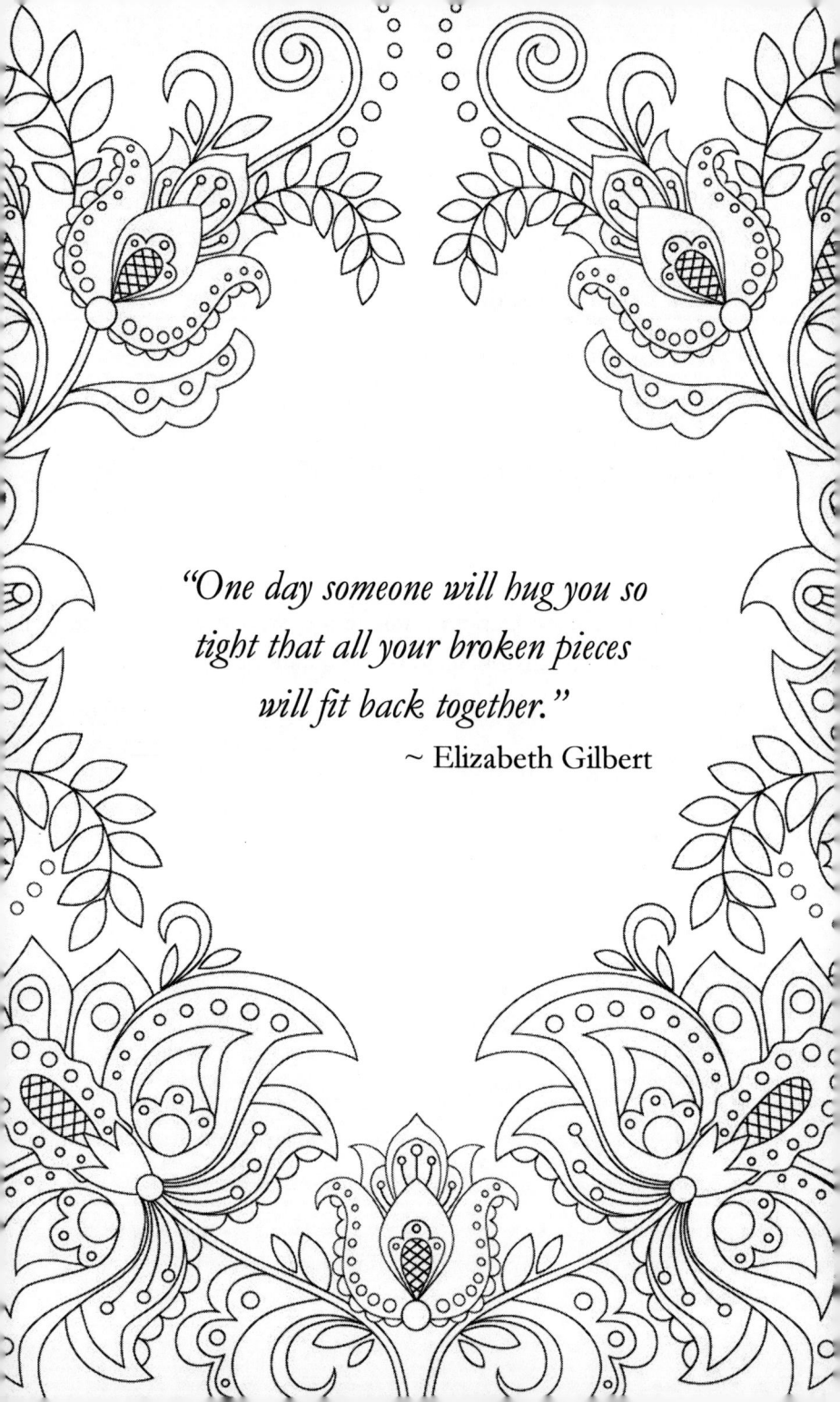

*"One day someone will hug you so
tight that all your broken pieces
will fit back together."*

~ Elizabeth Gilbert

Chapter 1

Your Inner Circle

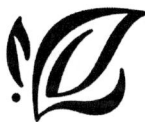

My broken moment manifested when I was 29, while I was living in Indianapolis, Indiana. It's hard to imagine that a single cold December day in 1999 could change my life, but it did. In the weeks leading up to that day, I had been feeling physically off. Energy low, muscles sore and achy, I would feel nauseous after every meal. I just didn't feel right. On this day in particular, my scalp was burning and throbbing more than usual in certain areas. The feeling had been gradually increasing, but I couldn't see it because it was on the back of my head. On this day, it was so annoying that I could not ignore it. I bought a hand-held mirror to see what was going on.

I was horrified.

Honestly, I couldn't believe what I was seeing. There were red, inflamed bald patches all over the back of my head. Big areas where my beautiful, thick black hair was now just gone. It was like a fire had scorched an area of a forest, and only a few trees and plants had survived. I started crying hysterically. I couldn't breathe. All I could do was fall to my knees and sob.

This broken moment opened the door to fear, worry, and panic. It was like the floor fell out from beneath me and I was in free fall. I was sinking and nothing made sense. I felt so alone and small. My confidence, self-worth and faith left me in that moment. I didn't know it then, but it would take ten painful years to revive them.

No one should have to suffer silently this way. We are complex beings who feel and heal. We are resilient and brave, but we do need others along the way, and they need us. But for me, this came a lot later.

After countless blood tests, biopsies, and specialist visits, I was diagnosed with an autoimmune disease that had no known cause.

After an extensive work-up, I was given a prescription for medication that made me more nauseous than my newly discovered dis-ease. (I refer to my illness as a dis-ease because I want the emphasis on the natural state of *ease* being imbalanced or disrupted. The idea is that when the body is out of balance or not at ease sickness happens, so our job is simply to bring back the ease.) Every time I had to take that little white pill, everything in my body revolted. It was such a visceral act of rebellion. I hated taking that fucking pill, and I felt betrayed by my body. My body was attacking itself.

After a couple of months of this inner struggle with taking that little white pill, I stopped. I'm not sure where that strength came from to make that decision, but because I was not getting answers about why I got sick, and the side effects made me feel worse than the original symptoms, I stopped.

Looking back, this was my first feeling of being guided. I will talk more about this feeling throughout the book. It's been a significant part of my healing. I felt a nudge, a strong gut feeling, and I trusted it, so I stopped. Later I became well acquainted with this voice/feeling. I didn't know it then, but this voice was my advocate, my biggest supporter, and it's always with me. It was me—but a wiser, calmer, grounded me. This voice doesn't let fear, worry, guilt or shame get the best of me. It stands up, and with strength, courage and bravery says, *There must be another way—we got this.*

I will never forget that feeling that washed over me when I was struggling with taking the little white pill. I felt as if the words bubbled up. *It's okay—if you don't want it, don't take it, it's okay.* I felt warmth and support first, then second thought, can I do that? The answer was of course, YES!

I stopped taking the little white pill. I continued with a blood test every other month, and I used a topical solution for my inflamed scalp. So many things still upset me about that whole situation, but this decision was made without regret. At this stage, I did not know how to access this calmer, wiser voice on a regular basis, so I would suffer for many years with fear and worry.

You, my darling, have an advocate, as well. It might be drowned out at the moment by both external and internal noise, but it's there. We all have a sacred place within us that guides and supports us unconditionally. You can call it your intuition or a gut feeling. When we get quiet and connect to that place, we feel guided. We're able to let things go to protect our energy and peace of mind, but when we're guided, we're also able to speak up and do what we feel is right. The outside noise, as well as our inner mental chatter fades, and we come from a place of knowing. Fear takes a back seat and our advocate stands with us and speaks through us. This practice of listening to your intuition is empowering. As I mentioned earlier, notice the things that catch your attention, even if they're faint and barely there. Take the time to be with things, people, environments that bring a sense of aliveness.

Ask Yourself …

- How strong is your inner circle?

- Are you able to share anything and everything with a few key people in your life? (You know, get support, give support, share your joys and your pains … everything.)

I love the term *inner circle* because for me it signifies a core group, or even just one or two people who take care of each other emotionally and mentally. I love the image of a circle because, when it comes to your inner circle, I think of everyone as being equal and connected. It can be your family … but only if you're able to fully open up to them. It can be friends you've gathered over the years. It can be a support group of any kind. There are no rules to this, except creating an environment of non-judgment, truth and unconditional support.

This was one of my mistakes that kept me sick, broken and unhappy for so many years. I did not share my pain about my dis-ease with another soul except my husband. My husband is a great guy, but he is not so great with deep talks or just being there as a listener. Like most men, he's a fixer. I have a problem; he wants to fix it. The emotional part is mostly a waste of time for him. Also, he's a doctor, so maybe because he's seen so much worse, and my condition was not terminal, he felt I should be fine. He didn't get it. He didn't know why I was so upset and couldn't move past what happened to me. The truth is, I didn't know why, either. I didn't share with him that I was scared about getting more sick and losing my vitality. He didn't know I was so fearful of losing all my hair and feeling ugly. He didn't know I felt broken and defective. He didn't know.

So for several years, I was alone with this sickness secret. Looking back, there were a couple of reasons I didn't share my pain. I didn't want to burden my family. I had lost my dad to lung cancer less than a year before; we as a family were devastated and heartbroken, and I did not want to add to their burden. I did not want anyone to worry about me. I also kept it quiet because I was embarrassed and ashamed of what happened to me. I could not even get myself to talk about it without sobbing uncontrollably.

Plus, there was a part of me that didn't want anyone to know I was broken. I liked presenting an image of having it all together. I was taught from a young age not to show weakness. My dis-ease made me vulnerable, and I was not comfortable with being vulnerable, so I kept it quiet. I had good friends, family—for God's sake, I have sisters! Really good ones, too. They would have done anything for me, but I could not get myself to utter words about my issue. My misstep was that I felt being vulnerable was a sign of weakness, and the last thing I wanted was for anyone to feel sorry for me. But vulnerability is what brings us together in a deeper way as human beings. We need people in order to add richness, love and light into our lives. We need people to expand our life. Being vulnerable releases us from guilt and/or shame.

It took me ten years after my diagnosis to tell my sisters and one of my dearest friends about my situation. I had done everything within my power to quietly heal myself, but it was not enough. For me to truly heal, I needed to share this experience with my people. I needed to be honest, vulnerable and get this last bit of stuck energy flowing. I remember so clearly the feeling that rushed through me after telling them. It was magical. Not magical like my hair grew back and I went right back to how I was before the diagnosis, but magical in the sense that I felt a stream of lightness, relief and okay-ness. Simply voicing my point of suffering without editing it released me of being tied to my condition.

I believe two major things happened for me when I shared my pain. One, someone listened and was a witness to my suffering and frustrations. I felt heard, and that alone can heal even the most wounded soul. Second, hearing myself telling my story gave me compassion toward my younger self. Knowing what I know now, I would have held that scared girl with open arms for as long as she needed. I would have let her cry and just be there with whatever she was experiencing—the good, the bad, and the ugly; all of it is beautiful because all of it is me. Being a witness and creating space for someone to heal is what I do in my Integrative Health Coaching Practice. My desire is to help my clients be compassionate toward themselves and accept all parts of their complex being. Each one of us is magnificent and unique. We were made that way.

Please, take a deep breath through the nose, hold at the top, and release.

There is a distinction I would like to make about sharing our stories as opposed to complaining about our issues again and again. There is a difference between being vulnerable by letting people in versus living in Victimville. That's why an inner circle is invaluable. Once you truthfully express (again, without editing) your unresolved stress, fear or pain point, you will feel different. Your energy will shift and lighten and your body will relax. Maybe hearing yourself talk will make the situation feel less scary. Maybe it will make it more important and valid. Or maybe just having someone listen helps you organize your feelings with more clarity. When you feel listened to and you speak your truth, big or small, healing happens. Once you get it out there, it no longer lives in your body. You can breathe more deeply.

However, unconscious complaining does not heal; it only grows that negative charge bigger and brings it closer to you. You can feel it in your body and mind.

It is important to share and release, but do it consciously with the right people; otherwise, it's like adding drops of gasoline to a fire. Sometimes people are so trapped in their stories that they don't even realize they're complaining. Their minds are constantly replaying the same tape, because they just can't let it go. This can be toxic. For a lot of people complaining is a way to socialize. Be aware of when you're doing this and change gears. Complaining unconsciously is being a victim and living from a space of blame and non-acceptance. When you are hooked to your story and unconsciously keep repeating it, you are reenacting what has happened to you and you are reliving it in your mind and body again and again. Your body has no idea if this happened 10 seconds ago or 10 years ago.

A good test to see whether you're in Victimville or in healing mode is to notice how you feel after the interaction. Whether it's a phone conversation or in person, a healing conversation will shift your energy and you will just feel better. Life is hard. We need people and people need us to navigate through this life. Sharing our struggles, pains, fears, worries, ideas, dreams and joys helps us become more human and increases our capacity to love. Whether you are the one creating space or the one speaking your truth, trust in the process and gather your people. Sometimes we are seeking advice and other times we just want to vent. Sometimes a solution comes—and sometimes it doesn't. We don't have to know the ending or have all the answers; we just speak from our heart and allow a space for others to speak theirs. These two acts have the power to not only heal us, but heal families, communities and the world.

Again, practice resisting the urge to be a casual complainer. Repeating our pain points or story to the wrong people does the opposite of healing; it gives your suffering legs and keeps it alive.

So pick your inner circle carefully.

Ask Yourself ...

- Do you have any secrets that are making you sick, mentally, emotionally, physically or spiritually?

- What are they? Write them down.

- Do you have someone you can share this with? Someone you trust and only wants the best for you?

If you have a broken moment or have been secretly suffering with something, it doesn't matter how long ago it happened. If you experience any negative emotion—fear, regret, shame, anger, sadness—when you think about it, it is still with you. Remember that your body and your subconscious mind do not know the difference between what is in the past and what is happening now. You must interrupt the story, let someone help you by being a witness to your pain and hold the space for you to release it.

What if you don't have a person like that in your life? Hire a professional. If your issue is around food or weight, hire a Health Coach. There are Life and Wellness Coaches popping up everywhere. We are all trained to listen for what needs to be healed. You'll know when you've found the right person because after a conversation with that person, you just feel better. Good coaches are trained to get your energy flowing. You should feel hopeful, maybe even inspired.

Listen, at the time when I was keeping my dis-ease quiet, I thought I was being strong and brave in my silent sufferings.

That's bullshit.

Let me share with you what was actually happening to me: with each passing day, the light in my eyes and the joy in my heart were fading. When darkness finds an opening and you do nothing to block it out, it moves in. Darkness came in and took residence. I was an excellent host to this houseguest. I fed it on a regular basis. It had all my attention and pretty much consumed me. I fanned its flame and kept its energy alive. I went to bed thinking about my bald patches and how unfair it was that I had to deal with this: "Why me? I don't want this! I just want to go back to the way things were." All these low energy thoughts put me in an unhealthy state as I drifted off to sleep. These vibrations would stay with me and I would wake up under a blanket of dread in the morning. And the whole process would start again.

See, all my negative thoughts had no place to go, because I didn't express them or release them in a healthy way. When you keep these things bottled up, they change you, because they influence how you think and feel, and what you do. They *change* you. You are loved. Allowing people to support you not only heals you, but deepens your bonds with your inner circle. Human beings need each other to feel worthy, to feel strong, to feel loved and to be enough. Decide never again to rob yourself and others of that gift. Your relationships will grow, and you will too. Having a strong inner circle will free you.

Share. Listen. Hold Space. *Be free.*

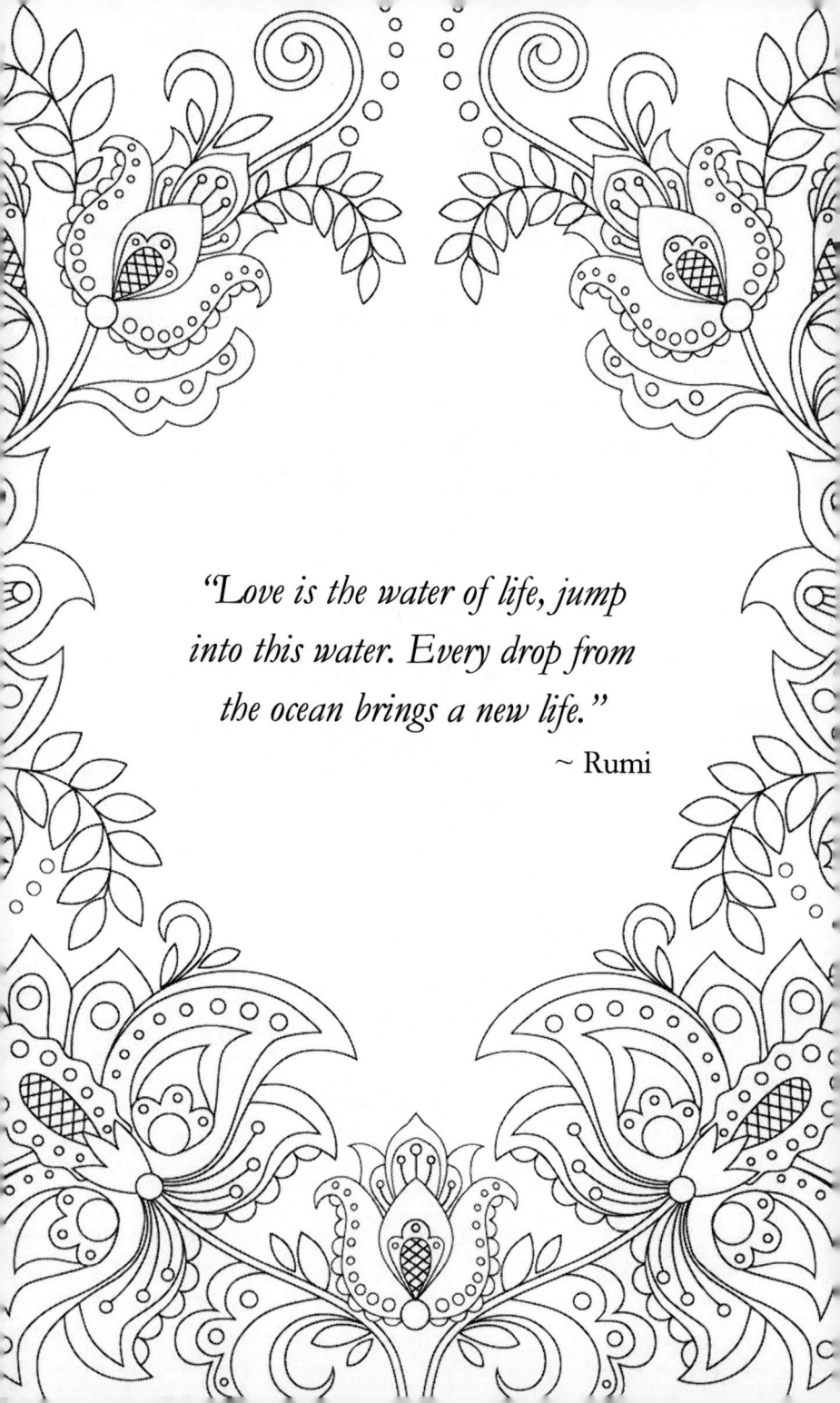

"Love is the water of life, jump
into this water. Every drop from
the ocean brings a new life."

~ Rumi

Chapter 2

Water

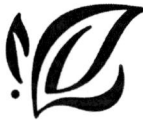

Everybody has got the memo on water, I get it, but *knowing* something and *doing* something are entirely different. I know some well-intentioned people who have not made this a habit. They drink some water if it comes up in conversation, or after they see an article on their newsfeed or on TV talking about its benefits, but then they stop. They don't make staying hydrated a part of their life.

As simple as it sounds, water is everything. If I get off track with how and what I want to eat, or I find myself craving sweet or salty snacks, the first thing I do is drink a full glass of water with a squeeze of fresh lemon juice. The water helps me reassess the situation, and I check back in. If I'm still peckish, the chances of me choosing a better food option are good.

It's one of the first things I start with in my private coaching program. Drinking enough water is an anchor. It gets you back on track. Try this for 21 days straight, no exceptions: Every morning heat up at least 12–15 ounces of filtered water to a comfortable warm temperature. Don't use the microwave; use a pot. Pour it in a glass, squeeze in some fresh lemon and do not walk away until you've finished it. All of it. Don't put it down and think you'll get back to it. You won't.

Getting this quantity of water with lemon first thing in the morning is major. Did you know that while you sleep, healing and recharging are happening? In a healthful environment, you stop eating three hours before bed and sleep at least seven hours a night. This means that by the time you have your warm lemon water in the morning, you have had roughly ten hours for your body to digest, heal, nourish and recharge. This also means when you take in that quantity of water first thing in the morning, your digestive system is getting rinsed and hydrated. The warmth of the water allows you to feel it move throughout your body, and it will make you feel so good to connect in this way every morning. My clients love this, too. For some, it has become a sacred ritual. If you do not like lemon water, apple cider vinegar is a great alternative. Just add one tablespoon to your 12-15 ounces of morning water. And if you don't like ACV, drink it plain. Water is life; just get some.

The more attention I give to how my body is responding to this radical act of self-care, the more I feel. Stay present while you are hydrating yourself. No matter how the previous day went, every morning I get a chance to start over and connect.

As far as the amount of water that you should drink, the rule of thumb is half your bodyweight in ounces. You can adjust that depending on how active you are, climate conditions, pregnancy, or any other health conditions. The amount recommended is just a guide. The most important thing you can do is see how increasing your water intake makes you feel. There are so many great benefits to drinking water, and I want you to experience them.

Replace any sugary (whether real sugar or fake) drinks with water. I know you know sodas (both regular and diet) are not healthy. However, I still see many people drinking sports or so-called vitamin drinks filled with not-so-healthy ingredients. It doesn't help that these products have high-profile athletes promoting them. Corporations spend millions of dollars branding these as health drinks; do not be played. Forget about what the packaging touts on the front, and look at the ingredients and nutritional facts on the back—the extra-small print.

I picked one up so I could go through the ingredient list with you. The first thing I always look at is serving size. The 28-ounce sports drink container I am looking at shows the serving size to be 12 ounces, so there are 2.5 servings per container.

The next thing I look at is sugar. Oh, sugar—you're sweet to the taste, but cause so much inflammation and weight gain. Cutting out sugar from my diet when I did my first 21-day cleanse helped me lose that last 5–8 pounds, which I had been sparring with for as long as I can remember. Sugar is in *everything*, and goes by many different names (56 different names, to be exact—sneaky. I have included a complete list of its aliases in the Appendix). According to the nutrition facts on the label, there are 21 grams of sugar in each serving—that's 5.25 teaspoons per serving. And remember: there are 2.5 servings. So that means this so-called healthy sports drink contains 13 teaspoons of sugar. Tell me, would you eat 13 teaspoons of sugar after an intense workout—or anytime, for that matter? I ask this because I have seen people at fitness clubs finish entire 28-ounce bottles at a time, and I honestly believe these people think they are being healthy by recovering electrolytes and hydrating.

Other ingredients in this particular sports drink are artificial colors, monopotassium phosphate, brominated vegetable oil (BVO), and other aliases of sugar (dextrose and sucrose). European labels contain warnings about artificial colors, but labels in the United States are not required to. Europe and other countries have actually banned BVO from products due to its health risks.

You don't have to be a scientist to see how this is going to end up. The ingredients speak for themselves. Sugar, artificial colors and flavors, some kind of emulsifier that contains endocrine disruptors, and more ingredients I can't spell or even say.

No, thank you. I opt out. I invite you to, as well. Drink water.

I also am a fan of pure coconut water to replenish electrolytes, and when you just need a little more. If you do choose to drink something else, put on those reading glasses if you must, and read the small print on the back.

A few tips:

As I mentioned, I drink a full glass of water first thing in the morning, and then sip throughout the day so I stay hydrated. During mealtimes, however, I have made it a habit to drink very little, if any. When we drink water while we eat, we are diluting the stomach acids and digestive enzymes, which are necessary for good digestion. Chew your food well and begin the digestion process with your saliva. By drinking enough water between meals, you will create a healthy environment for your food to breakdown, process nutrients and eliminate waste. This is what your digestive system is meant to do to keep you nourished, happy, and healthy.

Also, I prefer room temperature, warm, or hot water—never ice water. Your body uses up unnecessary energy to heat up the water for proper digestion. I used to take the digestive process for granted, but now I have come to learn how much energy it takes the body to assimilate our food, and I want to help it along. At restaurants, I always order water without ice.

If you get lemon with water while you're eating out, once you squeeze the lemon juice in, don't put the lemon itself into your water. You don't know where it's been rolling around, and organic lemons are expensive, so chances are these little guys have been sprayed and not washed.

And finally, my last little nugget: if you choose to have a cocktail or wine, remember to have a glass of water right after. One cocktail/wine to one glass of water. You will stay hydrated, and because of all the fluids, you will naturally drink less alcohol. In the morning, your body will thank you.

Ask Yourself …

- Are you drinking half your bodyweight in ounces of water?
- What tips from this chapter do you think you can incorporate?
- Do you think you can do it for 21 days?

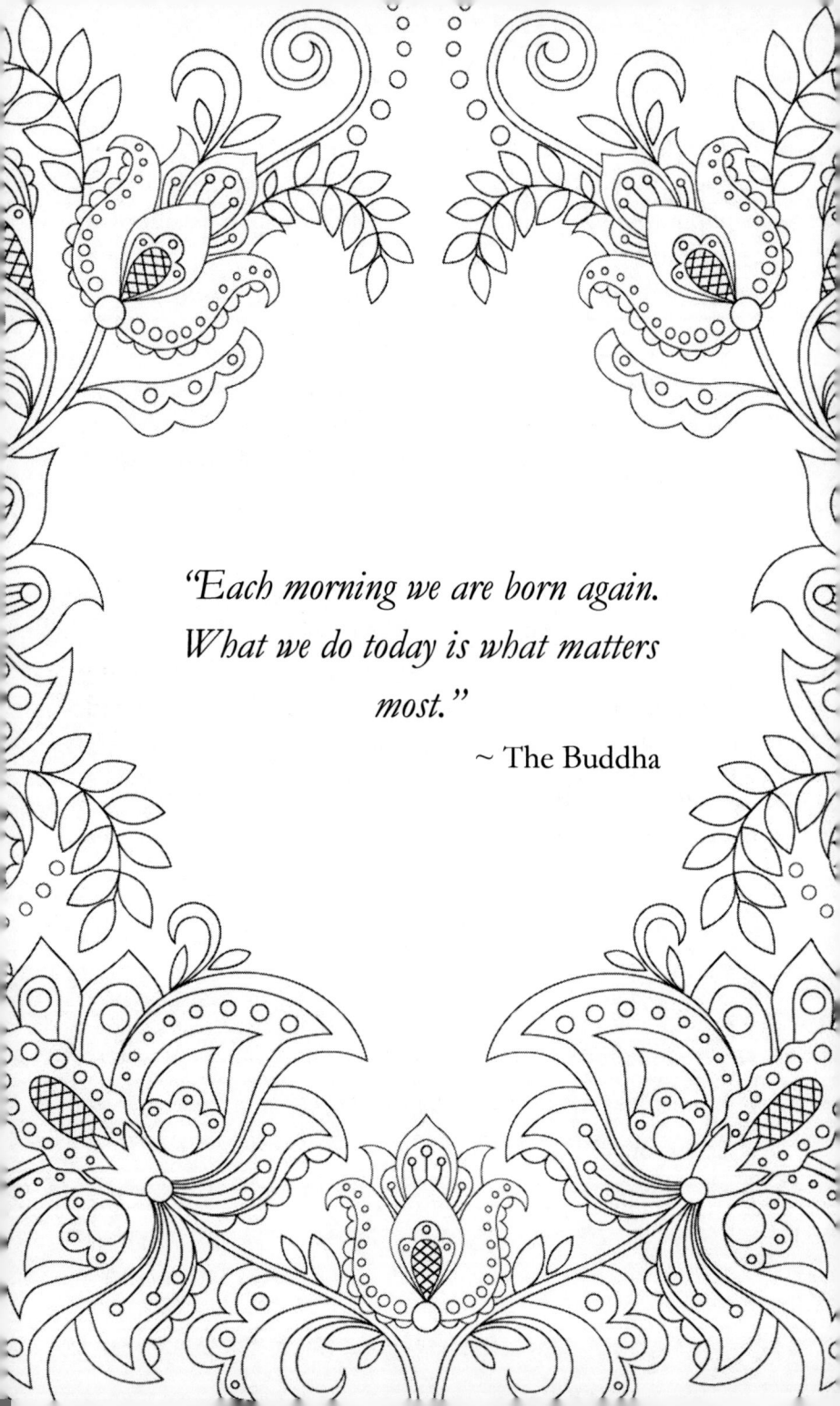

"Each morning we are born again.
What we do today is what matters
most."

~ The Buddha

Chapter 3

Sleep

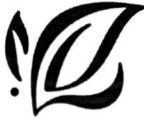

What can I say about sleep? *A lot.* Again, it sounds like a no-brainer, but so many people aren't getting enough. Sleep is one of those things—like water—that if you don't get enough, it can wreak havoc with your health and life goals. And I know that if you're reading this book, you either have a plan or you want one. You are not half-assing this living-with-vitality thing.

When we're not rested, we tend to reach for caffeine and sugary foods to get through the day. We crave foods that will give us quick energy; however, with that quick energy comes a commensurate crash. It's called credit-card energy—get the benefits now, but pay later. Without enough sleep, your focus will be on just trying to get through the day—forget about creating anything new. I'm not talking about a day here or there, when you were not able to get to bed on time or you had to wake up extra early for some reason. I'm talking about the daily habit of getting distracted by meaningless things like watching TV or being on the internet, and not getting the sleep you deserve.

That's right, you *deserve* to feel rested.

I know this first hand. One of my self-sabotaging habits was watching hours of mindless TV at night. I hate to admit this, but when the kids were younger, I valued my evening me time so intensely that I couldn't wait till dinner was done, the kitchen was clean, and the kids were in bed. For me, that was my time to do whatever I wanted. Because I'd spent the day doing everything for everyone else and being good with my diet (I don't use that word anymore, by the way), it meant I deserved to watch mindless reality shows and eat snacks I enjoyed. It was my time, period. I justified this mindset for a couple of years.

Then what do you think happened in the morning? I felt bad about what I ate. I felt bad about staying up too late because I was tired. I needed to work off the calories and I willed myself to be good. Being *good* meant working out hard, running for 45 to 60 minutes, and restricting what I ate (I don't use the word *restricting* anymore, either).

This doesn't sound bad, right? I was just being *healthy*; I was just being *good*. NO! This mindset was not serving my highest good or greatest joy. I became rigid and strict.

I was punishing myself. This was not sustainable or healthy. Most nights, I went back to doing the same thing. It was like there was a night *me* and a morning *me*, and if they'd gone to school together, they would never have been friends.

Take a deep breath through the nose, hold at the top, and release.

Most of us know the ways we self-sabotage, but we have no clue that this is a form of self-punishment, which we often justify in the name of being healthy or being good. If you have struggled with releasing extra weight, struggled with energy and feeling good in your body, I bet there is a lack of true self-love or self-care. When you instill those qualities and strive for them every day, guilt, punishment, feeling bad and self-sabotage will fade away.

Once I got this, it was no longer about being good or bad; it was about taking care of myself and loving myself enough to naturally do the right things. I interrupted the pattern and implemented new habits that felt good in the long-term. That felt in alignment with what I really wanted. Feeling good in the short-term is no substitution for long-term health and happiness. Now, when I wake up from a restful sleep, I am able to naturally make decisions that support my long-term health and wellness goals.

I'm betting you already know it's important to get high quality, sound sleep, and you don't need a list, or research or a big study done over several decades to prove that sleep is a Pillar for Health and Wholeness. It just is.

That's the thing with truth: it's always there and doesn't change. It's not new; the new part is something in you that has opened up to finally receive it and take action. I want you to get to know that feeling of truth within you and take action from that place, not because it's on a list, or because an expert told you, but because to know it will help you not only with health goals, but with your life.

Connecting to that place within is freedom, and we all have that ability. That's why phrases like *I've got a gut feeling* or *something doesn't feel right* are so common. All I want you to do is recognize for yourself that beautiful feeling of knowing. I call this *trusting in your truth*. If you, my darling, start following its thread, I promise you it will uncover the beauty that lies within you.

By now you might be thinking, *Wait, what happened? We were talking about getting enough sleep, and now we're talking about trusting in your truth?*

Stay with me, I'll get you there. Like a mobile phone that loses its charge, so do we. When you sleep, you recharge your mind, your body, and, depending on what you believe in, your spirit. Sleep plugs us in. Some believe that when we sleep, we plug back to Source, or to the divinity from which we come. When we sleep, we are pulled back to our true nature and are given the opportunity every morning to start fresh, so that when we wake, we have the clarity and strength to walk toward our dreams.

I want to repeat this: *we sleep to connect to our true nature so when we wake, we can walk toward our dreams.* When you feed yourself this kind of uninterrupted nourishment, you become the author of your life. By that, I don't mean that sleep will fix everything in your life. I am suggesting that when we get enough high-quality sleep, we have the energy and clarity to go after what we want. Every day, consciously or not, we are making decisions that support what we want, how we want to be in the world, and what we're going to do to get there. If we're not in the right frame of mind, it becomes extremely difficult to stay on the path.

I don't know about you, but when I'm tired, I can barely get through the day. (These are also very common phrases in our culture: *I'm surviving* or *I'm getting through the day.* Life is too precious to go through it with that attitude, isn't it?) We are the creators of our own lives. We are the authors of our own stories. How are we going to create and author with sleepy eyes, tired bodies, and foggy minds?

We can't.

So if you are not getting enough sleep and don't have a bedtime routine, make it happen. It will give you a clearer mind with which to make better decisions, which in turn will make you productive and healthful. When you rest your body at night, you will feel good about your day and look forward to getting a good night sleep, so you can start again. Maybe even jumping out of bed with excitement before your alarm clock goes off. (Too soon? I'm just saying it's possible …)

Some bedtime tips:

- Drink most of your water before the early evening so you don't interrupt your precious deep sleep by having to use the bathroom.

- Shut down all your technology at least an hour before bed. Lower the bright lights in your home at least three hours before bedtime, maybe light a few candles instead. The blue rays in lights and screens shut down melatonin production. Melatonin is produced by the body and is referred to as the sleep hormone. It tells your body that it's nighttime and it's time to go to bed.

- If you do use your computer, there is a free online program, f.lux.com, which removes blue light from your computer screen. Also, check if your phone or tablet has a night shift button. If not, you can cover your devices with a blue-blocking filter.

- Read something positive before bedtime, and when you rest your head on your pillow, go through your day and list three to five things you're grateful for.

- If you still have trouble calming your mind, then keep a notebook and pen by your bedside and write down all the things you have to do tomorrow. Write down anything you're anxious about not getting done. Write it all down, getting it out of your head and onto paper. This list will be there in the morning, so you can relax and get a good night sleep.

- Take a few deep cleansing breaths and allow the body to release and fully let go onto your bed.

- If you need an alarm clock, do not hit snooze when it goes off. Get up and stretch your entire body. Full body stretch. Set the tone for your day. You, my dear, are not a snoozer.

- As your feet touch the floor, offer thanks for a good sleep.

I love all the Pillars, and every single one of them is important. However, if you're feeling overwhelmed and finding it difficult to get a handle on where to start, then start here. Getting enough water and quality sleep are major, and will change your life. I go back to these two anchors again and again if I notice myself going back to old patterns, or in a direction I don't like. Water and sleep ... come back to them again and again.

Ask Yourself:

- Are you waking up rested and ready to go?

- If not, what can you start doing differently today?

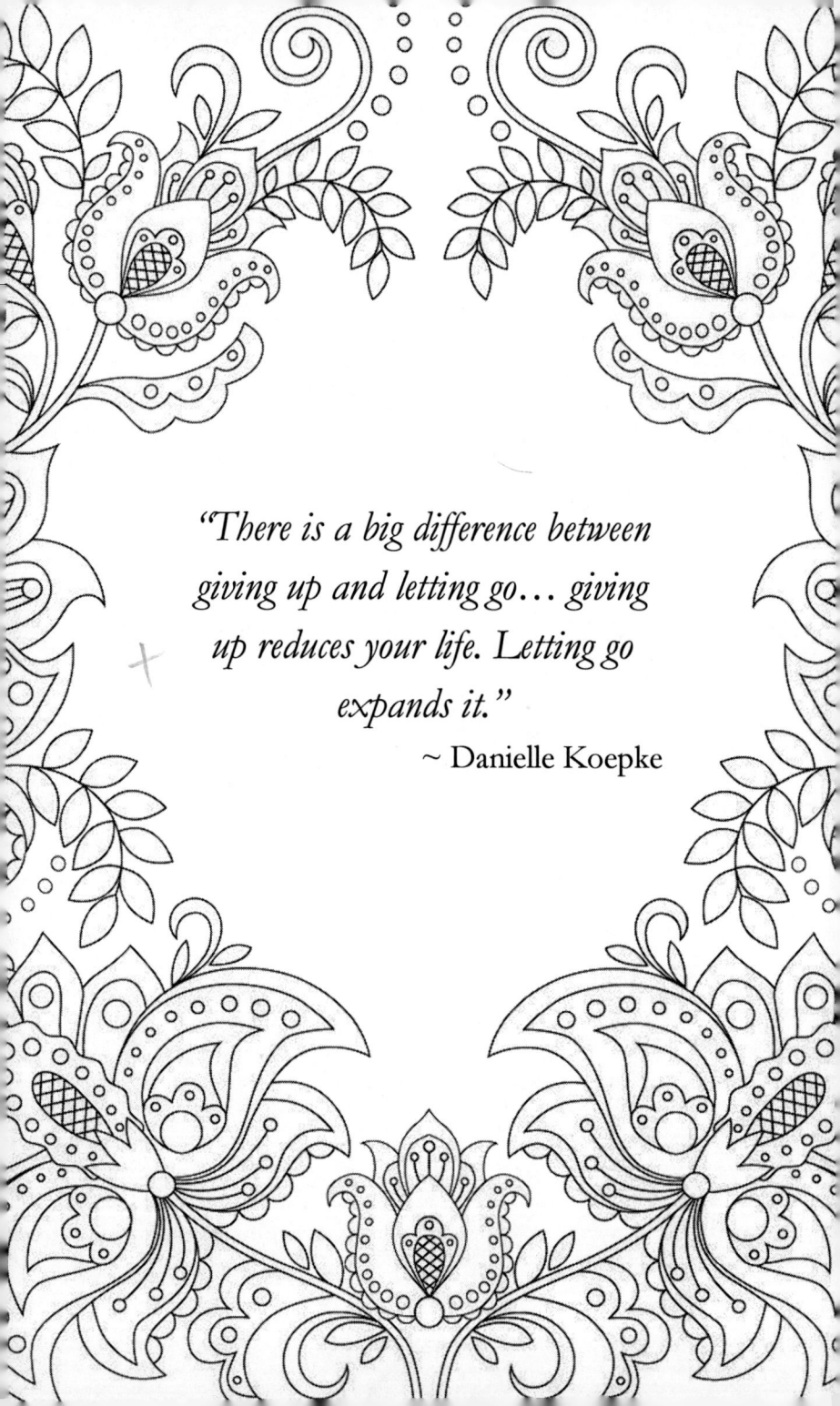

"There is a big difference between giving up and letting go… giving up reduces your life. Letting go expands it."

~ Danielle Koepke

Chapter 4

Movement

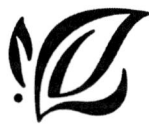

Water and sleep are anchors. When they are off, we are off. Come back again and again to make sure these anchors are set.

What happens when they become habits? Glad I asked! The answer is you *feel better*. You wake up without an alarm clock, you're ready for your day, you have energy and enthusiasm, and you *require* movement. You naturally want to do what feels right for your body, so you move. Exercise sometimes feels like a *have to*, but when you are hydrated and rested, you are pulled to move and it becomes a *want to*.

I have no set exercise plan for you. Everyone is different and has different preferences. So you get to pick. My only request is that, whatever it is, make it enjoyable and be consistent. You might love a good, hard, sweaty group fitness class, Zumba, running, cycling, yoga or hiking in the woods … it doesn't matter, just move. My sister swears by hula hooping. She loves it and does it any chance she gets. You might do better with people or alone. It's all good.

Also, don't be afraid to switch it up. When I was a runner, training for half marathons and a marathon in 2005, running was part of my identity: *Hi, I'm Rita, wife, mother of three, runner, grew up in California—and did I mention I'm a runner?* We all have identities that are part of our unique personality, but I know for me it took a while to admit running was no longer serving me. In fact, it was wearing me out. We are evolving beings, and change is part of this evolution. My point here is just listen to your body, and every so often check in and see how you feel. Does your choice of movement energize you? Or exhaust you? Your exercise or movement plan should add value and energy to your life, not drain you of your energy for the rest of the day. For most of us, our movement plan should be a part of our life, not something that consumes it.

After my diagnosis and my decision not to take those little white pills, I was on a mission to fix my body by myself. If I thought something was healthy, I did more of it. If salads were good, I would eat them twice a day every day. If cardio was good, I wouldn't miss a workout. We had a fitness center where I worked, so at lunchtime I would take group fitness classes. I was there every day.

My co-workers were avid runners, and before I knew it, I'd joined a running group. My husband was heavily into his residency program and studying for Boards at the time, so I spent a lot of time with my running group. After work, we would go on long runs. I signed up for races and half-marathons and immersed myself in the world of running.

At that time, I found comfort in running. The repetition of pounding the pavement cleared my mind, and I experienced a glimmer of relief from my usual stream of worry. It's like running tired out not only my legs, but my mind, too, so eventually all of me could rest. I was hooked.

I remember the first time I experienced this sense of relief, what I've come to call *the space*. I was running in my neighborhood during the fall. The weather was getting cooler, and leaves were falling and blowing in the wind. During that run something magical happened, I felt so alive and present. I felt so connected to the trees and the birds and the breeze. It's like we were all in sync and floating. No separation. No boundaries. Just connectedness, stillness, and I felt a burst of unconditional love.

Of course, the space faded, and the chatter in my mind and the fear in my heart returned, but it didn't matter. I had felt the possibility, and it has never left me. I ran every day to rendezvous with this space, and every day I would encounter that feeling at some level. Some days the pull was stronger and I felt alive; other days it would just brush by me, leaving its scent. I lived for that space, because other times during the day felt crowded and painful.

Looking back, I was suffering. Suffering is when you are living in the past with regret, guilt, bitterness, shame or in the future with worry and fear. Suffering is when you don't accept the *Now*, when you are not living in the present moment.

Eckhart Tolle taught me these concepts in his books *The Power of Now* and *A New Earth*. Do yourself a favor and read them. The concepts are timeless and the lessons are pure gold.

Looking back, suffering for me meant wanting the past to change. I remember wanting nothing more than to go back to the way I was, pre-dis-ease. That desire was so powerful that it robbed me of the present. As Tolle teaches in his books, interviews, and videos, the present is the only place that your life is happening. A beautiful day was lost on me; I couldn't have seen it during those times if it had hit me on the head. Delicious food with the company of family and friends became a burden, because they got in the way of my pity party for one.

As I mentioned earlier, I did not have a strong inner circle, and not having one stunted my healing. As a result, I led two separate lives. With people, I was an imitation of what I previously was. Alone, I was mostly sad and stuck in my story. Both versions were negative and toxic.

Running brought me back to a place of feeling whole again, and not separate or fractured. I wanted to know what this feeling was and how I could bring more of it to the rest of my life, so I ran. Now I refer to this space as sacred, and I've become a serious student of experiencing it. I read books, enrolled in programs and workshops that taught all about health, wellness, healing, meditation, spirituality and happiness. That little space not only had a feeling, but sometimes a gentle voice. I would hear her faintly saying, *It's going to be okay. You're okay. I'm here.*

Please, take a deep breath through the nose, hold at the top, and release.

One day while I was training for a marathon, a running mate casually mentioned that she had found yoga helpful and that I should try it. Our long runs were always on Saturday or Sunday, so the following Monday, without much thought, I went to my first yoga class.

I remember that class vividly. It was at a gym that had been a department store, and the yoga class took place in the old shoe section. There were none of the fancy yoga/spa amenities that I have since experienced. Just a bunch of people with mats and a desire to stretch, strengthen and heal something.

Grace entered for me in two ways: the first had been my friend casually mentioning her yoga experience, and the second was the teacher who was there on that first day. Her words, her presence and her kindness felt like home. The yoga teacher led us through a slow vinyasa flow, and by the end of class, my body was buzzing. The space expanded in savasana, which is the final resting pose after every yoga class.

I was a regular in this Monday night class, and six months later, I signed up for a teacher training program. Now I teach at the same place I was introduced to this beautiful, healing practice. Connie, my first yoga teacher, still teaches there, too. We have become friends.

I tell you this story because I want you to find something that not only strengthens and tones your body, but I want you to find something that opens you up and connects you to your wholeness. Walking in nature can do this. Dancing can do this. So many beautiful things can come from this place of feeling whole again. You start feeling guided. The right people, situations, books or anything else you desire—and some things you didn't even know you wanted—will start coming your way. It feels like a coincidence or synchronicity, but it's not. It's what the Zen masters call *living in flow.*

Why am I telling you this? Stay with me; I'll circle back to movement.

During my over-exercising, running-four-to-six-miles-a-day days, I was an *active couch potato*—a well-intended exerciser who exercises and then sits for long periods of time. It's that mindset of, "I just worked out or just ran five miles, and now it's okay to sit down, watch TV, and chill for hours."

Because I linked being exhausted to being physically active and strong, I felt pretty accomplished, and I believed I had earned the right to relax and take it easy the rest of the day. Little did I know that sitting for long periods of time was canceling out all the benefits from running. I was also frustrated about not being able to lose any weight. In fact, I put on a few pounds.

Turns out, the sit-on-my-butt card I gifted myself after an intense run slowed down my metabolism, while increasing both blood glucose and blood pressure. Marc Hamilton, Ph.D., professor and director of the inactivity physiology department at Pennington Biomedical Research Center, puts it this way: "Sitting for an extended period of time causes your body to shut down at the metabolic level. When your muscles are immobile, your circulation slows, so you're using less blood sugar and you're burning less fat." Basically, the body goes into fat storage mode.

Due to my autoimmune situation, running would have me laid out on the couch for a couple of hours a day. Thinking back, I sincerely thought I was being healthy. I identified with being a runner and I desperately wanted my health back to the way it was BD (before dis-ease); consequently, I was willing to bust my ass for it. But ironically, my intense bursts of exercise were making things worse in more than one way.

When I think about what I put my body through and how hard my poor body continuously worked for me, it makes me sad. I did not take one second to heed my body's call for recovery and rest. I was in the *no pain, no gain* mindset: if I wanted to get my health back and be skinny, I had to work my butt off; only lazy people rested or did the easy stuff. Running was for hard-core health conscious people, and I wanted to be in that club. Little did I realize that I was unconsciously abusing my body. Running fanned the flames of my inflammation and my dis-ease progressed. I was confused and frustrated that I was feeling worse. I experienced flu-like symptoms of achiness, fatigue, chills, low energy and brain fog on a regular basis. What really started to worry me was my inability to concentrate, my constant irritability, and the cloud of anxiety and worry that never left me.

This went on for a couple of years. Each day my light dimmed, my world got smaller, and I became more isolated. The lesson for me was that I did not need to work so hard at working out to get healthy and feel strong. I did not have to compete with my old self, or what I was once able to do. My body is forever changing, and therefore I must make adjustments. Our bodies are constantly giving us feedback, and to gain real health and vitality, we must listen.

I do not regret running for all those years. Training and completing a marathon will always be a time that I hold special. Running was my first conscious experience of the space. That space of connectedness and alertness. That space of being completely in my body.

But what I discovered after chasing my health for four hours and 33 minutes, step by step completing a marathon, was that *more* does not mean *better*. While I honor people who have the capacity to do it and to benefit from their regimen, busting my ass for health is no longer part of my belief system. Listening to our bodies is the best we can ever do. Now I practice yoga and walk in nature to nourish that part of me. The vehicle changed, but the journey of seeking sacred space continues.

Don't be afraid to change and don't over-identify with being one thing. You, my darling, are complex, evolving, and magnificent. Your body is speaking to you all the time. When you start to listen, your health and vitality will improve. The vitality of your body is in direct correlation to how connected you are to it.

Ask Yourself …

- Does your movement plan give you energy?

- How has your movement plan changed in the last year, five years, and ten years?

- If you have changed, then when you look back, how does it make you feel?

- What are your favorite ways to get moving? Write down everything you have ever loved since you were a child.

- Do you enjoy group classes or flying solo?

- What time of day works best for you?

- What are you committed to do more of on a consistent basis?

- Lastly, share your plan with your inner circle and maybe buddy up. Accountability and support will keep you on track, plus it's just more fun.

I don't know where I read this, but I couldn't agree more—exercise should be a celebration of what your body can do. Not a punishment for what you ate. Human beings are designed to move, and the healthiest people in the world are upright and moving most of their day. So let's get off our chairs and/or couches and move!

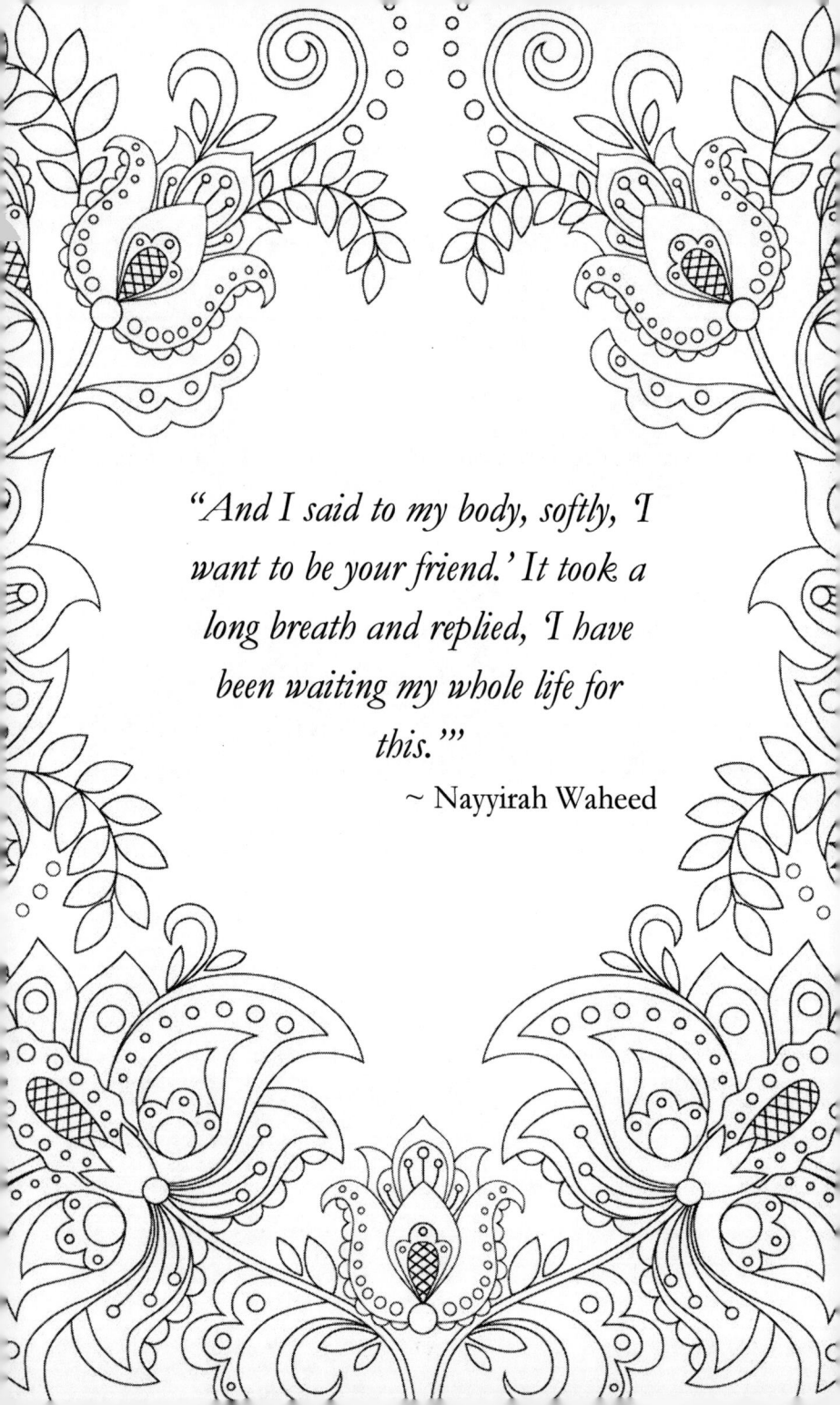

"And I said to my body, softly, 'I want to be your friend.' It took a long breath and replied, 'I have been waiting my whole life for this.'"

~ Nayyirah Waheed

Chapter 5

Stress Management

 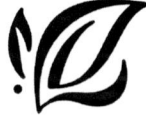

Let's face it: life is stressful. There is no way around it. If you go to school, have a job, have a family, have friends, or own your own business, then you have more than likely bumped up against stress.

The sense of a lack of control in a situation contributes to feeling stressed. Most adults are pretty familiar with this feeling. Stress or feeling anxious is a normal part of everyday life for most of us. It's even expected in some situations: if you're not stressed, you're not doing enough. This is the school of thought most of us have grown up with.

The inconsistency is that most of us also believe stress is bad. We are all trying to get rid of it. We all crave a stress-free life, yet if we are not stressed, we don't feel productive—and that gives us stress.

Is it just me, or are we all crazy?

I don't believe all stress is bad. I believe stress can be a great activator to do incredible things. Stress can spark ideas, even create the urgency to make significant decisions that improve the quality of your life in an instant. However, it is true that if stress runs your show, it can lead to unhealthy choices and/or sickness.

But you have a choice when it comes to stress.

I didn't always believe this; in fact, stress and I had a volatile relationship for decades, but we finally came to an understanding. Here it is: I will acknowledge stress, but not be dragged around by it. Stress now offers me information, and I have the option to use it … or not. Stress is my servant, and it helps me get things done in a timely way.

Sounds good, right? To understand how I came to this, let me share what I previously believed.

I don't remember being a stressed-out kid; intense, perhaps, but not stressed. Schoolwork, getting good grades and having good times were all part of my daily world, and I took them in stride. Stress is not natural for younger children, because they are masters at being present and living each moment as it unfolds. I don't even remember the word *stress* being thrown around much. As we grow, things happen to us or to people we care about, and we lose that ability to come from a clean space. Most of us begin to *live* in the past or future, and that's where suffering or stress comes in; we're not actually living when we run the tapes of the past or the future.

Once I got this message—I mean, *really* got it—I was able to clearly see where I was getting tripped up and missing chunks of my life. The *Now* is the only place life is happening. Tolle wrote about this beautifully in *The Power of Now*, and Deepak Chopra talks about this in his books and lectures. In fact, Chopra says the only moment that matters is the one happening now. The people who are most important are the people you are with now. Once we practice living in the present, our stress has the potential to vanish. I'm not saying the present moment cannot have stress; I'm just saying a large percentage of the stress we carry is created by the anger or hurt which accompany thoughts about the past and/or future. I have noticed this in myself and others: stress comes from regret, pain, or grief of the past, or it can come from worry, anxiety or fear for the future. The present is usually a safe place. We just forget to live there because our minds are time traveling.

Our belief systems, the thoughts we think, the words we repeat again and again can create our reality. I want to give you a personal example. As I mentioned, I was not generally a stressed kid, but there was always one thing I was petrified of, and that was contracting a disease. I'm not sure how this fear entered, but I remember during my middle and high-school years, whenever I would learn about an illness at school or on the news, I was secretly scared I had it. I didn't talk about it to anyone; I would just think and worry about it when I was alone. When I was with people, I would get distracted and forget about it, till I learned about some other illness.

The other memory I have from a young age is of my mom's thinning hair. As far back as I can remember, my mother had extremely thin hair. She never would talk about it or act alarmed by her situation—but I was. I was sad for her and fearful for myself because I thought I was going to get whatever this was. That feeling never stayed front and center for long; my family was pretty involved in our community and with a family business, and with the busyness of the days and years, we kept moving forward.

But as I watched my mom's hair get thinner and thinner, I would notice the hairs on my own brush. I would notice—and suffer over—how many strands of hair I would lose in the drain when I washed my hair. I would feel so sad when I would notice my mom spending so much time trying to spread out her thin hair with a fine-tooth comb to cover her scalp. I had a head of thick, beautiful black hair, and I felt so guilty for having it.

I remember having two distinct feelings about my mom's hair. First, a longing to be able to take some of my hair and give it to her. Next, fear of losing my own. This became a regular thought pattern every time I combed or washed my hair. I was caught in the worry of future pain of fear for myself and past pain of regret for my mom's loss. Being caught in this type of pain led to many years of suffering. I could not fully enjoy what I had, for fear of losing it. Even though I was functioning, and for the most part a pretty joyful, enthusiastic person, every time I washed or combed my hair, the thought of my mom's hair and losing my own hair crept in. It would fade once I was distracted with something else, but that thought was never far away.

I'm not sure how many hours, days, months or even years of energy I wasted, but this pain took up residence in my mind and settled in, eventually becoming a part of me.

Most women I know have experienced a relationship like this with their bodies. We are never happy with what we look like. Years pass by. When we look back at ourselves in photos from our twenties, thirties, forties, fifties and beyond, we wonder why didn't we wear more dresses, short skirts, or two-piece bathing suits. Why didn't we just enjoy our bodies? Why were we so hard on ourselves?

I have no scientific proof of what I'm about to tell you, but I believe it to be true with all my heart. As I mentioned earlier, our thoughts become our reality. I made myself sick. My fear of having some awful disease and losing my hair like my mom ignited my dis-ease. I never spoke about this fear with anyone. Not my sisters or friends or my mom. I talked to no one. This shadow lived in me. Our thoughts have power, and continuous thoughts that don't have a way to be released eventually manifest. Energy goes where attention flows.

Not long after I got married, my parents came to visit me and I noticed my mom's hair was painfully thinner. She kept nervously trying to fix it, and probably could sense that I noticed. I felt so bad that she had to deal with this, almost like it was happening to me. But isn't that how we feel pain when our loved ones are suffering? She never complained. Even though I could tell by her nervous energy that the suffering was taking up immense space in her heart and mind, my mom never allowed her pain to get in the way of taking care of her family. I wanted her to talk about it. I wanted to know how it started, what it was, and if she was okay. But I didn't ask, and she didn't share, either. So we both avoided it and talked about everything else.

The next morning they left, and while I was showering, I started to cry. Shower cries were a safe place for me to let go and feel. That night I came up with a plan to gather my loose strands and make a wig for my mom. Maybe I could ask my sisters to do the same, I thought. I didn't even know if this was something that was possible, but I didn't care, I needed to do something. I did this for weeks, and it was a big mess. I couldn't keep the strands from tangling, and every time I would see the bag of hair I was collecting, I would feel awful about all the hair I was losing. It was not a healthy situation.

Eventually, I came up with a better solution for my mom's issue, but here is the takeaway: I was consumed with fear and worry. I took it in. This statement is everything; I'm going to say it again: *I took it in.* My body did not know whether this was happening to me or someone else, because the negative emotion around it was so strong. I took it in. My thoughts were running a non-stop loop of this *I'm gonna get sick* song.

I did not realize the full extent of the damage that I was causing, because I still managed to enjoy parts of my life. I worked at a job I loved, was around great people, and enjoyed my time. I thought I was handling it. But the truth was that the repetition of the negative loop I had created for so long attached to a strong emotion, becoming a limiting belief.

Beliefs are powerful. They can drive us to set the world on fire and do amazing things, but negative beliefs can limit us and keep us stuck. This belief about getting sick, inheriting my mom's issue, coupled with overwhelming sadness, led to that winter day in 1999. I made myself sick. Again, can I prove this? No, but I know it in my heart, and I have made peace with it.

Through my healing process and from writing this book, I finally took the opportunity to ask my sisters about their experience with our mom's thinning hair, and how they took it in growing up. All of them were aware our mom's hair was thin. They did feel compassion for her, and sympathy that she had to deal with it, but for the most part, they just accepted it. That was just our mom. Because she never complained or talked about it, it was a non-issue for them. They also never had thoughts growing up about illness or inheriting our mom's thinning hair situation.

I find that fascinating. My sisters did not take it in, and the daughter who did (me) was the one who eventually manifested the dis-ease. It was no accident. It has taken me 17 years since that winter day to own this conclusion. Our thoughts continually direct our lives. Our thoughts—which lead to emotions, which lead to behaviors, which then mold the belief system that is the foundation and lens through which we see everything.

For me this was a hard lesson, but there was a silver lining: the opposite of this emotional loop is also true. You have the power to redirect negative to positive, and change your life with just your thoughts and the power of positive energy (emotions). My constant, unnecessary, negative thoughts led to unnecessary stress, which made me sick. This is what stress does if it is not managed. Once we know how to use it to our advantage, stress is no longer the enemy. It becomes our ally. Once you recognize and bring awareness to stress, you, my darling, can transmute it to pure energy and make it serve you.

Interested in learning how to do this?

Please, take a deep breath through the nose, hold at the top, and release.

I have read that we have on average 60,000 thoughts a day. They say 80% are negative, and 95% of those negative thoughts are repetitive. That's a lot of negative, destructive energy out there. This energy does not just die once a thought is internally expressed—it vibrates, and will tend to attract similar energy, possibly even the exact thing you have been stressing about. I don't think you want that; I know I didn't. Understanding this can be life-changing if you take the time to work through it.

Here is how I healed my mind, my heart and eventually my body, and how you can, too:

- Notice the negative, repetitive thoughts you think. Actually take a pause and notice what you think about.

- Write them down—all of them. It might take you a few days to pinpoint the repetitive ones, but it's important to take the time. Don't sugar-coat them. If you can capture the exact thought, word for word, that would be helpful.

- Notice what emotion is tied to the thought. Write that down, too.

- Once you have captured enough to work with, pick a day when you are feeling good about yourself and look over the list. It's important to make sure it's a day you feel optimistic, because we want your true self to call bullshit on those fear-based thoughts. If you can't muster enough good feelings, ask a trusted friend to help you with this part.

- For each thought, ask, "Is this true? Do I know this for sure?" No buts, sometimes, or excuses—simply True or Not True.

- For absolutely True, you will need to deal with it, and either accept or change. Take some time to know how you feel about it, and get some help if you need to.

- I am more interested in the Not True, repetitive, negative, bullshit thoughts. If you're not sure, keep asking the question: "Is this true?"

- Then write the reasons that it is not true. Give yourself evidence that it is not true.

- If Not True, rewrite the thought to a neutral or positive thought.

Here is an example of the bullshit negativity that was running me for so many years:

Negative repetitive thought: *My body has failed me. I am broken.*

Emotion: *Angry, sad and ashamed.*

Was it true? *NO!*

What *was* true: *After the diagnosis, I gave birth to three beautiful, healthy children. This body allows me to experience the world, connect with people every day, practice and teach yoga. My body is brilliant and works hard for me to obtain balance and good health.*

True Statements: *My body is a miracle. I am healing. I am a miracle.*

These True Statements are called affirmations. This type of work, given some patience and time, will shift your limiting beliefs and bring in healing. In the beginning, it didn't feel right to jump all the way over to *I am so healthy*, because I was dealing with a real health issue. I had big bald patches on my scalp and I felt sick. I knew I couldn't just pretend at this stage, so instead I acknowledged my body for the miracle it is, and I would repeat every day, "I am healing, I am healing, I am healing." Meanwhile, I would take small steps in learning about nutrition, changing my diet, learning about how stress affects the body, talking to various types of doctors, both western and eastern trained. My go-to's were the ones who were trained in both. I required a doctor who both understood the science and respected the natural healing properties of the body.

Depending on how ingrained each thought is, this may take some time. Be patient and trust that it is working on a subconscious level. That's why it is so hard to make real, lasting changes. We may say, "Okay, I'm going to eat right, exercise daily, change jobs, and start a new business," or something as simple as, "I'm just going to take care of myself." But I have noticed that, for myself and my clients, until we deal with our limiting beliefs, real, lasting change is not possible. So if you are having trouble sticking to your changes, please, take the time to acknowledge your negative thoughts and go through the questions above until you come up with empowering statements.

Once you have your new beliefs, find a quiet time, preferably in the morning before the day gets rolling, and read to yourself the revised positive or neutral messages. Take long deep breaths, allow the words to rinse over you. Louise Hay is the queen of affirmations, and her book *You Can Heal Your Life* is where I discovered them. Making this my daily practice has been a blessing. At that time, I had no idea how it worked or if it would work for me, but I didn't care—I needed something. Let me be honest, at first, I did not believe those statements—my ingrained negative beliefs felt more real—but after a month of doing these every day, I owned them fully. I added:

- *I am healthy and whole.*

- *I am full of vibrant energy and strength.*

- *I love my body* [this was a big one for me].

These statements have become new beliefs for me, and are ingrained even more deeply than the false negative ones I acquired along the way. I *am* all these things, and no person or situation can change that without my permission. The freedom and peace of mind that come from this type of practice is priceless. Try it for yourself and witness your life unfolding. Your thoughts are shaping your life anyway—you might as well do it consciously.

Running, as I mentioned, was my first experience in being in *the space* and being present. But practicing yoga integrated it into my nervous system, and became a source of daily stress relief and discovery. I know yoga is not for everyone. I get it. What I am asking of you is to find something that relieves you of negative self-talk and brings you into the present. Spending time alone is important to access this part. The biggest complaint I hear from my clients when I ask them to create a stress-management plan is, "I don't have the time." My answer is always, "Let's make some time, it's important."

Here's a simple 15–20 minute routine that includes clearing your mind, getting focused, and attracting good, nurturing energy. This exercise pulls it all together:

- If you wake up with a head full of to-dos and concerns, the first thing to do is to write it all down.

- Write down the things that are bothering you, write down your to-do list, write down anything that is occupying space in your mind. Don't worry about grammar or spelling or being poetic, just get it out. I've heard this called a brain dump.

- Then once you get all the noise on paper, write down three things you are grateful for. The simpler the better.

- Next, take a look at your paper, circle or put a check on the things you are going to get to today. Then scan your gratitude list. Put your paper on the side, close your eyes, and do the Buddha belly breaths I introduced earlier. Deep belly breaths soothe your nervous system, slow everything down, and help you be more focused and clear.

- Next, in your mind, bring up the three things you wrote down that you are grateful for. Bring them up one at a time and allow the feeling of gratitude to wash over you.

- Lastly, repeat the positive affirmations. Remember, you might not believe them 100% just yet, but no worries ... it's coming.

My hope is that you take some time and practice these simple techniques. Be open to the process and maybe even feel something. Even a small shift is worth exploration.

Besides yoga, journaling, breathing exercises, gratitude and meditation, walking amongst the trees, birds and open sky is also a great way to reconnect and feel grounded. Hiking brings me to that quiet space of knowing who I am. I'm not sure how it happens, but nature does that for me. It gives me the opportunity to reconnect with my true self. All the nonsense drops away, and I'm left with the things that give my life meaning and purpose. I love yoga and walking because they fulfill four of the Pillars: movement, stress management, connecting to something bigger and finally, a pocket of joy. I typically walk alone and get that time for myself to *just be*. As a yoga teacher and an Integrative Health Coach, it's important for me to reconnect with myself every day. I would not be able to serve and be fully present for my clients, to give them the attention and energy they need if I didn't take time for myself.

We all need to recharge and replenish our energy. I always hear women talk about *me time* and *taking care of themselves*, but I'm not sure most women know how to do this. No judgment here; I know when you have dedicated your life to taking care of others, it's challenging to start looking after yourself. My clients tell me that taking the time to do a few things for themselves every day feels wasteful or less important than doing the things on their to-do lists. I have also heard women say they feel guilty, and that they're just too busy with all the little fires that need to be put out throughout the day.

These feelings are normal. However, if you continue to make the time to do what you say you are going to do for yourself, these feelings will pass and you will make self-care a priority. All the other things will get done, and maybe some of the things on your list will feel less important. Our priorities start to shift and we start feeling in control of our day and of our future. One thing I encourage is that whatever stress management techniques you choose, do them at least three or four times a week. Doing them every single day for a month is even better. Making them a habit is key. Not just when you've had enough or you're frustrated with your situation, but also when things are good. Build up your reserves, so that in any given situation, you are centered and grounded.

Ask Yourself …

- What can you commit to doing every day to make sure you are managing your stress, reconnecting to your truth and clearing out negative thoughts?

Possible ideas:

- Identifying and shifting limiting beliefs.

- Journaling, brain dump.

- Listing your to-do's so you don't have to carry them around in your mind.

- Breathing exercise.

- Gratitude exercise.

- Yoga.

- Meditation.

- Walking in nature.

Remember, do what fills you up. Make it your practice, and let it be something that offers you a lasting feeling of wellness, not just a short-term fix. There is a difference. For example, if you're an emotional eater, a piece of your favorite dessert might cover up the stress, and you'll feel better for a bit. However, if guilt follows, having that piece of cake is creating suffering, not peace. Stress management techniques are best when they are aligned with your health and wellness long-term goals.

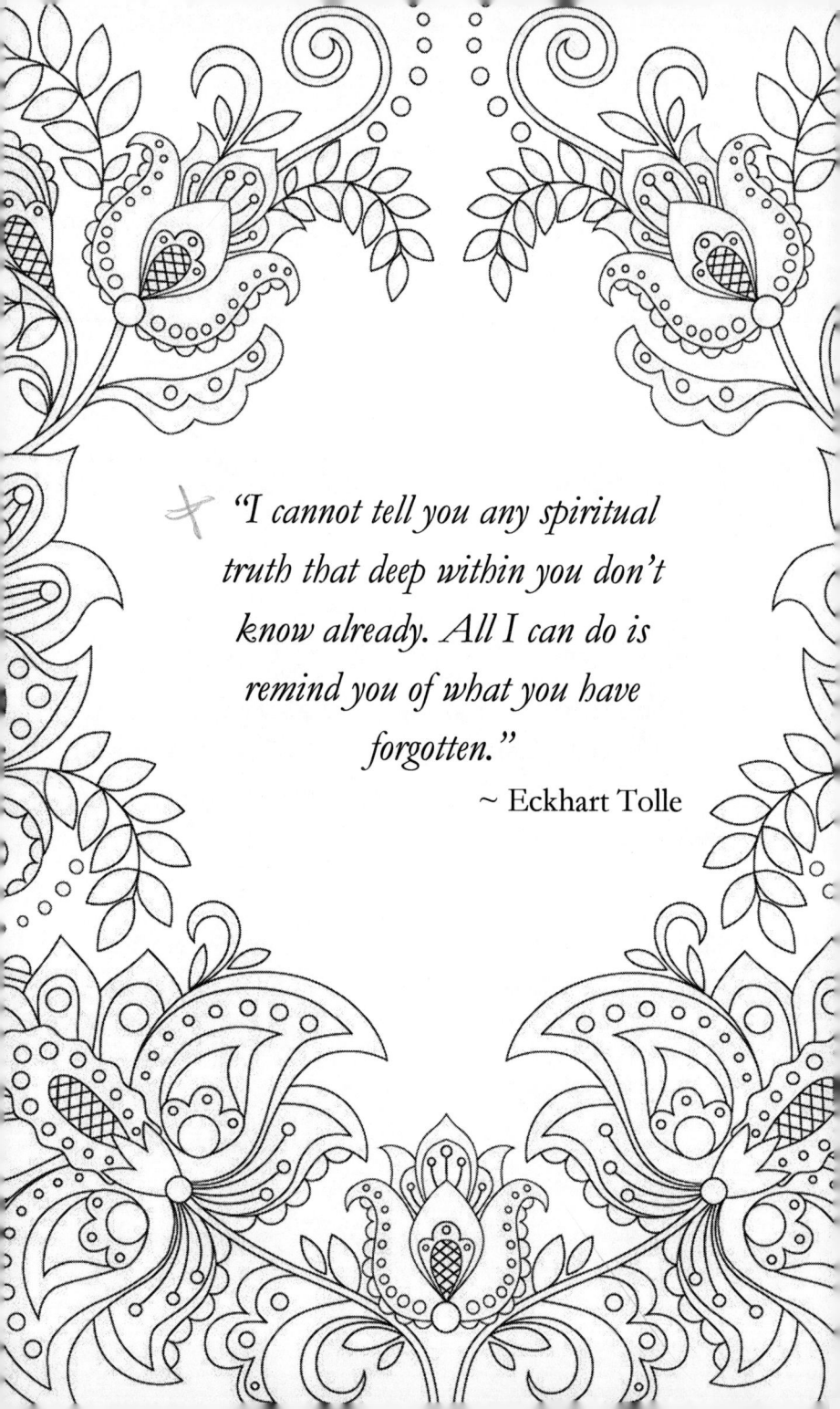

"I cannot tell you any spiritual truth that deep within you don't know already. All I can do is remind you of what you have forgotten."

~ Eckhart Tolle

Chapter 6

Connection to Something Bigger

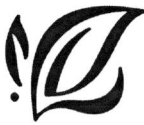

Do you ever look back and think how fearless and confident you were as a kid, teenager or young adult? Then something happened along the way and it broke your spirit. Maybe it even caused you to close up your wings and start playing it safe. It could be a disappointment or the loss of a job or loved one. It could be an unhappy marriage or an illness. We just get smaller and more fearful about our lives.

During these times, it's easy to check out. You may even rationalize your withdrawal by saying: *I was good. I did all the right things. I didn't deserve this; I did my part and life screwed me. Life hurt me, and I am going to protect myself.* What happens over time, though, is that in the process of protecting ourselves and putting up walls, we also block the good stuff from coming in. We stunt our growth and our potential.

I wholeheartedly agree that life can be hard. But life is also a gift. *You* are a gift. And as a gift, life is something that must be unwrapped and revealed as we go. Being open and curious about life will bring aliveness and beauty to our experience.

Please, don't get me wrong here, I know people—maybe even you—have real challenges and have been through it. Honestly, I have not met a soul over the age of 25 who hasn't.

When I was diagnosed and feeling quite ill, both physically and emotionally, I experienced a kind of shrinking. I was so stuck in the story of my sickness and getting back to the way I was, I was unable to receive the moment to moment blessings that come with life. A beautiful day no longer lit me up. Delicious foods and spending time with family and friends became a burden. Negative thoughts of my dis-ease were front and center and ran my life.

It feels weird to write this, but I think feeling sorry for myself and being a victim were the only things that gave me comfort. My sorrow and I became great bed buddies. My thoughts all stemmed from fear. I did not understand the power of thoughts. I did not understand that I was not my thoughts. These thoughts—and the fear they created—ran my life. When I woke up in the morning, there they were, and they were still running through my head as I laid my head on the pillow at night.

These were my thoughts:

- I am going to die.

- I'm not going to be able to have children.

- I am going bald.

- I hate my body.

- I am unlovable.

- My body has betrayed me.

- I feel defective and broken.

- I want to go back to the way things were before this thing interrupted my life.

- I am not enough.

- Why the fuck is this happening to me?

I did not want this dis-ease, so all I gave it was negative energy, hoping and praying it would just go away. I think that's why I didn't tell anyone, because if I had, that would have made it more real.

Thus began my double life. Around people, I would muster up a version of what I was, and alone, I would marinate my sadness. My poor husband never knew who he was going to get—pity-party Rita or the watered-down version. He would try to comfort me by telling me it wasn't a big deal, and would call me Telly Savalas. For him, it was a way to bring light; for me it was a little insensitive.

(Right? Seriously, referencing a bald guy?!).

I was not ready to joke about my condition. How could I be a miserable, hopeless victim if I was laughing about it? No, no, I took this depression thing very seriously! I had a no-laughing policy. As I mentioned earlier, I found solace in running, and for the first time I started to earnestly pray.

I grew up in a religious family with lots of deities and traditions. I didn't really understand why we did some of the things we did, but I would do them because they were expected. Even after I got married, I set up an altar in my home like most Indian households have, designated for lighting a diva (candle) and for prayer. I never felt authentic doing the ritual, because I didn't know what I was doing. I knew I needed to do something, and so I began to pray.

One prayer I became attached to was in a small booklet, which contained the Hanuman Chalisa. This prayer had 40 verses, and I would chant it daily, sometimes three or four times a day. The 25th verse was of particular interest to me:

Nase rog harai sab peera,

Japat nirantar Hanumant beera.

Which translates to: Disease will be ended, all pains will be gone, when a devotee continuously repeats Hanuman the Brave's name.

Sign me up. That is all I wanted. I wanted my dis-ease and pain gone. Just like running and yoga class, chanting these verses, listening to them in the car, gave me comfort and opened up a space for me to rest. I didn't know it then, but I was gathering my tools to one day heal and be free. I didn't know it then, but being *broken* became my biggest gift. Back then, those spaces were my lifeline. The moments were small and elusive, but so real. I became a seeker.

In 2000, we moved here to Columbus, Ohio, where my husband joined a practice. That year I got pregnant and felt so grateful for this blessing. One life-changing thing I noticed while I was pregnant was that I started feeling better. My scalp did not burn as much, and after the first trimester, I no longer felt nauseous after I ate a meal. I also stopped losing copious amounts of hair. I felt good. I was not completely back to being myself, but I felt some relief.

After giving birth and having this beautiful child, my thoughts drifted away from my own experience and turned to my mother. Over the course of being diagnosed and keeping my condition a secret, I would say my capacity to receive and give love narrowed in all areas except one. I thought about my mom a lot. How did she deal with the thinning of her hair while raising five children, having limited income, having no real voice in a stressful marriage? I love my dad, but he wasn't the easiest person to live with. My mother's role was to cook, clean, work at the business, and serve. She did it with love and devotion.

The questions I kept spinning were:

- How did she keep her spirits up?

- Was she also leading a double life?

- How did she not lose her shit?

- How come I was so weak?

After I gave birth, for the first time I saw my mother as a woman, a human being with emotions, wants, and maybe even dreams. I felt so much compassion, admiration and love for this woman. In this space, I wanted to know her pain and help her any way I could. One day, when we were on the phone, I found an opening and went for it—I mustered enough courage to ask her about her hair. "Mommy, are you okay about your hair?" She paused. There was complete silence, and I held that space for her. She finally said softly, "I don't like it, but what can I do?"

That was all I needed to hear. Strength and confidence like I'd never known before rushed through me. I was going to help her find peace with this, no matter what. I had never felt this type of certainty or sense of mission as I did in that moment.

The word that comes to mind is Dharma. The concept of Dharma is taught in both the Hindu and Buddhist religions. The Merriam-Webster dictionary defines it as an individual's duty fulfilled by observance of custom or law, and also is defined as conformity to one's duty and nature. In the teachings of yoga, Dharma refers to your work or purpose. Dharma is what your soul signed up for. The interesting part is that your happiness is tied to your Dharma. So it's about you, your work, your happiness, and also how it serves your family, community—maybe even the world. I knew this was my Dharma—to help my mom find a solution. I was doing my Dharma, and when you're doing your Dharma, you are guided and nothing gets in your way. I had already researched a place in Northern California that makes prosthetic full hairpieces with the best quality human hair, for people dealing with alopecia or cancer. I asked her how she felt about checking it out with me and potentially getting a wig. To my surprise, and without hesitation, she said *yes*.

My heart opened and my belly relaxed. She said *yes!* I wanted to take that yes and do somersaults. It made me so happy that she said yes. During this time, I had a beautiful, healthy one-year-old, and was six months pregnant with my second. I flew to Los Angeles with my son, dropped him off with my sister-in-law and brother, picked up my mom, and we hopped on a flight to San Francisco. My mom was beyond nervous and anxious. She had no idea what to expect, but her known pain was more painful than the unknown. That is a great place for change to happen.

For the first time, I experienced what it felt like to just hold space for someone who was suffering. I didn't care if she cried, didn't talk, or even yelled at me. I was just there for her. I remember being so acutely aware of her energy, and for once I was not consumed with my own shit. I loved the aliveness that I was experiencing. I was listening, not anticipating. I was breathing slowly and felt clear. I was completely in my body, with a heightened alertness and an open heart that was motivated by pure service.

Being fully present with my mom freed up my cluttered mind, and just being there for another human being sparked my interest to come to this place of service. When I hitched on to a higher energy through pure service, I created more power, more love, more kindness, more faith and fear left me. I desired to take up residence in this new space I had discovered.

Some people look to religion for this, and that's great. As long as you feel more peaceful, clear and connected, it's all good. For me, creating a space for others has become a passion. Creating that space for others, whether I'm teaching yoga or health coaching, helps me connect again and again to that feeling I had with my mom. In yoga, I talk about *the space* all the time. At the end of each class, I invite students to linger in the space that they created with their attention and breath, and allow it to settle. I'm always surprised when students thank me, because holding that space lifts me up again and again.

Ask Yourself ...

- Have you ever felt so much certainty about doing something, no matter what obstacles came your way?

- Have you ever felt guided?

- If so, when?

- What did that feel like?

- How was your energy?

- Did fear play any part?

When a space like this opens up, magic ensues. I am forever a seeker of this kind of space, and I hope you will be, as well. Resting in the space is personally healing, and holding a space for others heals them, too. In this space, you will feel whole, alive and content. Nothing lacking or broken, you'll find that you are perfectly imperfect ... and that is perfect.

Please, take a deep breath through the nose, hold at the top, and release.

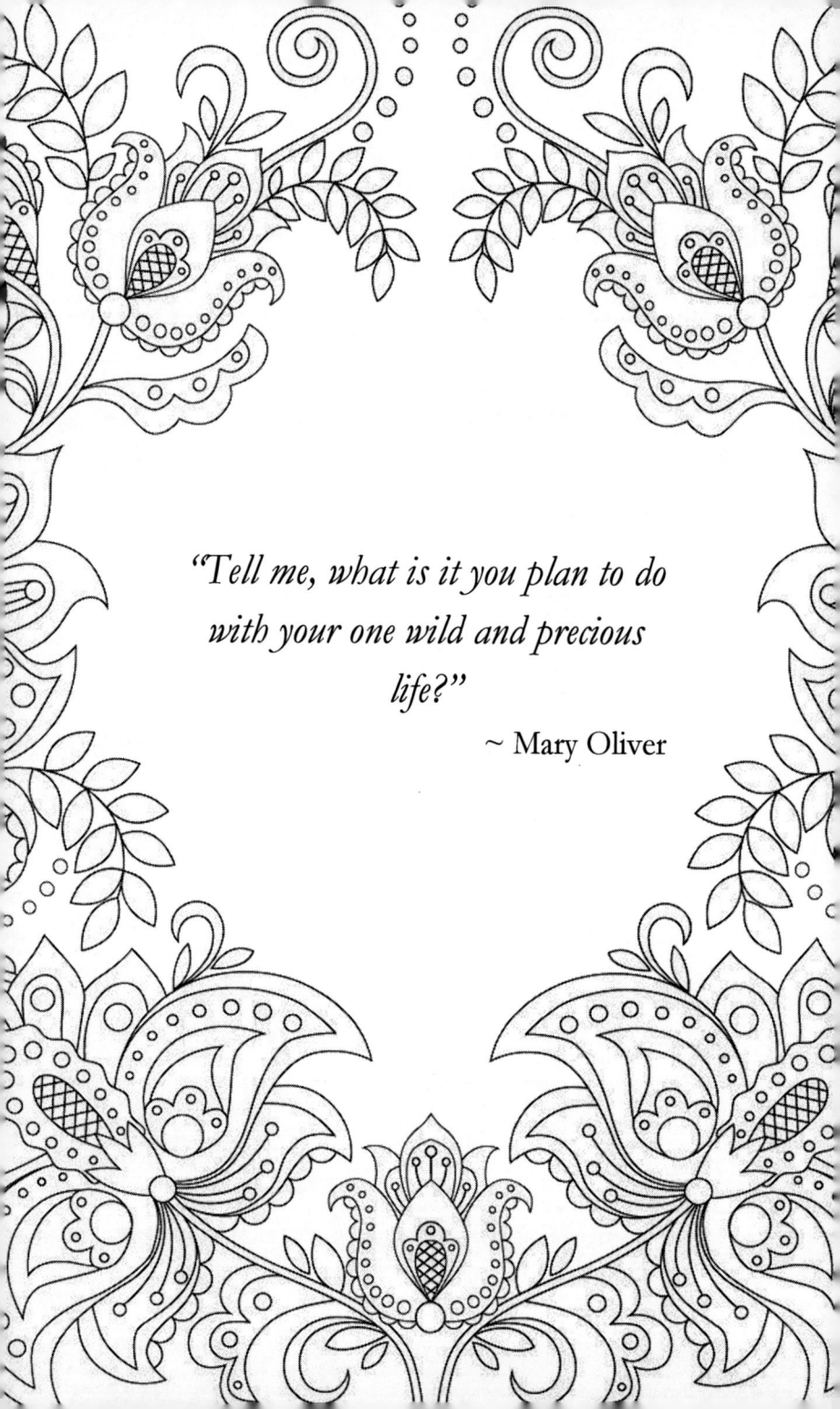

"Tell me, what is it you plan to do with your one wild and precious life?"

~ Mary Oliver

Chapter 7

Pockets of Joy

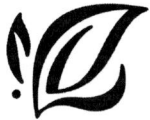

Connecting to something bigger helps you to connect to yourself. From 2001 through the end of 2004, I gave birth to three healthy, beautiful babies. Being pregnant taught me a lot about the healing properties of the body. Our bodies are truly magnificent, given the chance. It was almost as if my body sent a memo to my mind which read: *I know you have been running the show for a while, but now a new life is being grown, and we (my body's healing properties, or Self with a capital S) are taking over. We are in charge. You can relax.*

So my small, fear-filled self surrendered and listened to what my body needed. I cared for my body more during pregnancy than any other time. Fed it whole, nutrient-dense foods. Drank plenty of water. Filled my mind with beautiful books on self-growth, healing and spirituality. I made sure to rest, but also moved more. It was during my pregnancies that I started appreciating long walks. I felt connected to my body and to everything around me. I remember going for walks late in the evenings, and feeling so connected to the trees, the sky, the sounds and the smells. All my senses felt heightened, and I enjoyed the clarity that heightened awareness gave my mind. I didn't know it then, but I was healing and I was creating a new track for my mind to play. This track was abundant, peaceful and compassionate. My small mind could not make what happened to me okay. My small mind could not accept it and forget about letting it go. No way—it needed a reason and it wanted to go back to the way I was. My small mind kept me stuck.

I want to be very clear about what suffering is. The Buddhists speak a lot about suffering, and it was not until I understood their definition that I was able to break free from the cycle that suffering causes. Suffering, as described by the Buddha, does not necessarily mean grave physical pain, but rather the mental suffering we undergo by holding onto things or people or an idea of what life should be like. The true nature of life is impermanent, yet we cling to our lives, our loved ones, and even things with an intensity that will bring what is called Dukkha. Dukkha is the experience of non-acceptance, and of holding on to a picture of what we once had, or think we should have. This is the gap where I suffered. However, once a space opened up for me to feel the loving hand of being connected and guided, it shifted.

When I feel connected, I accept it all. The good and the bad.

When I am connected, there is no going back to the way things were; there is only now.

When I am connected, my mind has clarity to find solutions and heal what I can.

When I am connected, I feel empowered.

When I am connected, I feel grateful for this body and all it allows me to see, be and do. I feel gratitude and unconditional acceptance for this body.

When I am connected, I feel so much compassion for my younger self. So many years of worry and guilt and the insatiable need to get back to the way I was. To be completely honest, I had thought, "This kind of thing happens to *other* people," and "Why me?"

When I'm connected, I ask a different question—what can I learn here? What is the lesson? And why *not* me?

When I am connected, I trust in sharing my struggles.

When I am connected, I heal.

When I connect to something bigger or to my bigger Self, there is no "I'll be happy when …" or "My life will start when …" There is you and me, and there is this moment. I don't know you, but I love you. You are loved. This is the feeling of being connected.

Ask Yourself …

- Are there areas in your life where you feel stuck? If so, what are they?

- Are there areas in your life that you have not accepted, that you feel bad about having to deal with?

- Are there areas of your life you know you need to change, but you spend more time thinking about why a thing happened than doing something about it?

- What is keeping you paralyzed?

- What do you need?

- What do you want?

Please, do not waste another moment running these negative tracks. They only attract more suffering and rob you of your birthright, which is joy, love and growth. Please hear me when I say that you did not deserve whatever happened to you. I am so deeply sorry for the pain it has caused you. You are not broken or defective, and should not be embarrassed about your struggle. As an Integrative Health Coach, this is one of the main ways I help people heal and get healthy and happy. As I mentioned earlier, people need a witness to their sadness and pain. As a coach, I am trained to get to the true sadness and support my client to let go and heal. From my own experience, it was in the active listening and presence of another human being that I healed. It is the feeling I had when I traveled with my mom to face her decades of suffering. When you connect to something bigger, you connect to your higher Self, and in that place you can find lasting peace, contentment, and even joy.

Connecting to something bigger doesn't have to be a religious or spiritual experience. Connecting to something bigger can be through your life's work, mission or passions.

The point is, there comes a time for us to experience happiness, and it has to be about something bigger.

I would love to tell you that once you experience this space, this stillness, this bliss, you are healed and done. Magic wand, you are enlightened. Done and done. Unfortunately, it doesn't work that way. Once the opening happens, it is our job to continue the journey. It's up to us to move toward that space and open it up. It's up to us to gradually release anything holding us back. The good news is that even if you feel too overwhelmed to make any significant changes, that space will never close. It will wait until you are ready. Some days you might feel the pull a little more than others, but it never goes away.

One way I stay connected to my true Self is by having a daily practice of gratitude. Being grateful is good for everyone, but this is especially useful for someone who is always expecting the other shoe to drop. If you naturally live in an anxious, stressed place, rewiring your brain to look for the good stuff will shift your energy. Being grateful every day and actively looking for things, people, and experiences I can appreciate keeps me at a healthier state of mind. Your mind is like a garden, and if you do not tend to your thoughts, weeds will take over. The best thing about creating this energy is that it will attract more of the same. This is not new. Countless books, spiritual teachers, self-growth teachers and gurus have talked about having an *attitude of gratitude*, yet, for some reason, people don't do it. Perhaps, as I mentioned in the beginning of the book, they think it's too simple, or that they already know about it, so they don't do it.

Not you, though. You know better, and as Maya Angelou says, *when you know better, you do better.*

Please, take a deep breath through the nose, hold at the top, and release.

I talked about bringing in gratitude under the Stress Management Pillar, but it's just as powerful a practice when used to Connect to Something Bigger. Every morning or before you go to bed think about three things that you are grateful for. The simpler the better. I love being thankful for the big things—my family, friends and good health—but I have found that looking for new things, no matter how simple, actually trains your brain to naturally look for more good stuff.

I read once that the human mind is like Velcro for negativity and like Teflon for positivity. Having a daily practice of gratitude changes this. We develop new pathways for searching out the good and letting the bad slide right off. Gratitude is the highest form of well-being. Being grateful puts you in a beautiful healing state. Your mind slows down and clarity comes in. Truth hits you in a more deliberate way. It doesn't just pass by; you take it in. The more I pay attention to these truths outside of me, the more I connect to my own truth. My own true nature. My intuition grows, and I feel pulled toward more of the same.

In flow, life feels effortless. The right information, people, experiences, and books come your way. At first, you think things happen by chance, or what a coincidence, but then you come to know it's because you are living in flow. A simple space or spark wakes you up to the magnificence of life. The awakening feels more like a recognition of what we have always known. Life sometimes has a way of covering it up, but I believe that the truth never dies. Once we get quiet, pay attention and connect to our true nature, our path unfolds. We are like plants that change our direction to face the sun. When we listen to our own truth, we turn effortlessly toward what lights us up.

Gratitude unlocks the fullness of life. It turns what we have into enough.

Once you discover these beautiful still spaces and/or your energy shifts, you might find yourself less interested in busy activities that once filled your days. This is not an accident or a phase; feelings of aliveness are clues to what lights us up. Our job is to follow them, and they will bring more joy, peace and love to our lives. Tapping into your truth and aliveness is an amazing journey that varies for everyone. Our path is as unique as we are. No two paths unfold in exactly the same way.

Unfortunately for most of us, our path to this place begins with pain, loss and/or dis-ease. The experience, if we let it, has a way of getting to the depths of our being. This jolt has the potential to wake us up to our true nature and heal us in such a way that we will never be the same.

After my diagnosis, running, walking in nature, chanting, yoga, meditation, and breathing exercises were all portals. These activities gave my relentless mind a break that allowed me to enter a safe space of presence. As I returned there again and again, I was able to notice and appreciate what was in front of me. I would seek out things that brought me back to my truth or brought me some joy or lightness.

As I mentioned, gratitude played a huge part in shifting my energy. To this day, it is a part of my daily practice, and I teach and share this with my yoga students and health coaching clients. Gratitude brought the joy back. Having fun and laughing is so healing and good for the soul. It is our job to bring it in. We have the power to bring lightness, joy and laughter in every moment … take it. When I teach my yoga classes, I take having fun very seriously. I want the students to leave with a sense of lightness and joy in their hearts. It's contagious; they then share it with whomever they encounter. I have noticed that the person who comes to class is different from the person who leaves.

When you start feeling better from working on the other Pillars, you will naturally want to bring in the joy. It is your nature, your birthright. Fill your days with as much laughter and joy as you can, there is no limit. I challenge myself to make a stranger laugh while I'm at the grocery store, or post office, or at the airport. I'm there; I might as well have fun. Stop saving your fun side. Unleash it and more will come. Just like love, compassion and kindness, it is abundant.

Ask Yourself …

- If you had two hours for yourself, what fun thing would you do?

- What would your perfect day be like?

- If you had an entire weekend to yourself, what would you do?

- I am most relaxed when I …?

- I feel most alive when I …?

- I have the most fun when …?

- Time flies when …?

- I feel most energized when …?

- I am most myself, living my truth when …?

Look over your answers and pick three things that you really love to do and, along with practicing gratitude, do those three things every day. Yes, every day. I call these Pockets of Joy. Bring into your day things that authentically bring you joy, peace of mind, and hopefully, some fun.

I use the word happiness, but my favorite word is joy, because happiness might come from something external, but joy is an inside job. Instead of waiting for the right time, like when you're on a beach with a cocktail in your hand, make a decision to create small pockets throughout your day. Thread them into your days and they will become a part of your life. Stop waiting. No, really—stop waiting for the right time, place, person, situation for you to give yourself permission to be happy. Joy doesn't just happen. It is a decision, and we can make it every day.

Just like I am asking you to do, I took time to figure out what things made me come alive, and I did them every day. A lot of my attention and energy went into doing things that gave me long-term joy, contentment, aliveness and a sense of pleasure.

Again, I emphasize long-term, because that big piece of chocolate cake, or four hours binge-watching Netflix, or surfing the black hole known as the internet might sound like a good way to "treat yourself" or "relax," but these things leave me feeling—for lack of a technical term—yucky. Empty, just not good. Listening to music, dancing, taking a bath or a long shower, a cup of tea or coffee, cooking, hanging out with my family and friends, trying new restaurants, traveling, reading a book—these all bring me joy. Just like gratitude, pockets of joy can be small. Seek them out and do them often. You are worth taking the time for, and your soul will thank you.

Oh, one more thing on this: don't fall into the trap of thinking that, in order to connect, you have to have an *Eat, Pray, Love* experience. One year traveling the world alone is fantastic if that's something you really want to do, but you can spark your flame with small, beautiful experiences practiced every day.

Even though no two paths are the same, it's no coincidence that breathing exercises like yoga, tai chi, qigong, walking in nature and meditation have helped so many people find peace, clarity and purpose. All of these activities quiet the mind. When the mind quiets, aliveness, intuition, and grace enter, and we become present. Some people discover this when they dance, paint, listen to music, cook, take a long, scenic drive, garden, or even clean their house. Our job is simply to pay attention to the feeling. If you are not sure or can't come up with anything, try a yoga class, or get out there in nature and just be. Become a seeker of what lights you up. Even the faintest of light or sensation is worth exploring. Your truth wants to be revealed. With a little attention and daily practice, it will grow, and so will you.

Give it a go, the journey will be worth it. I promise. Start today.

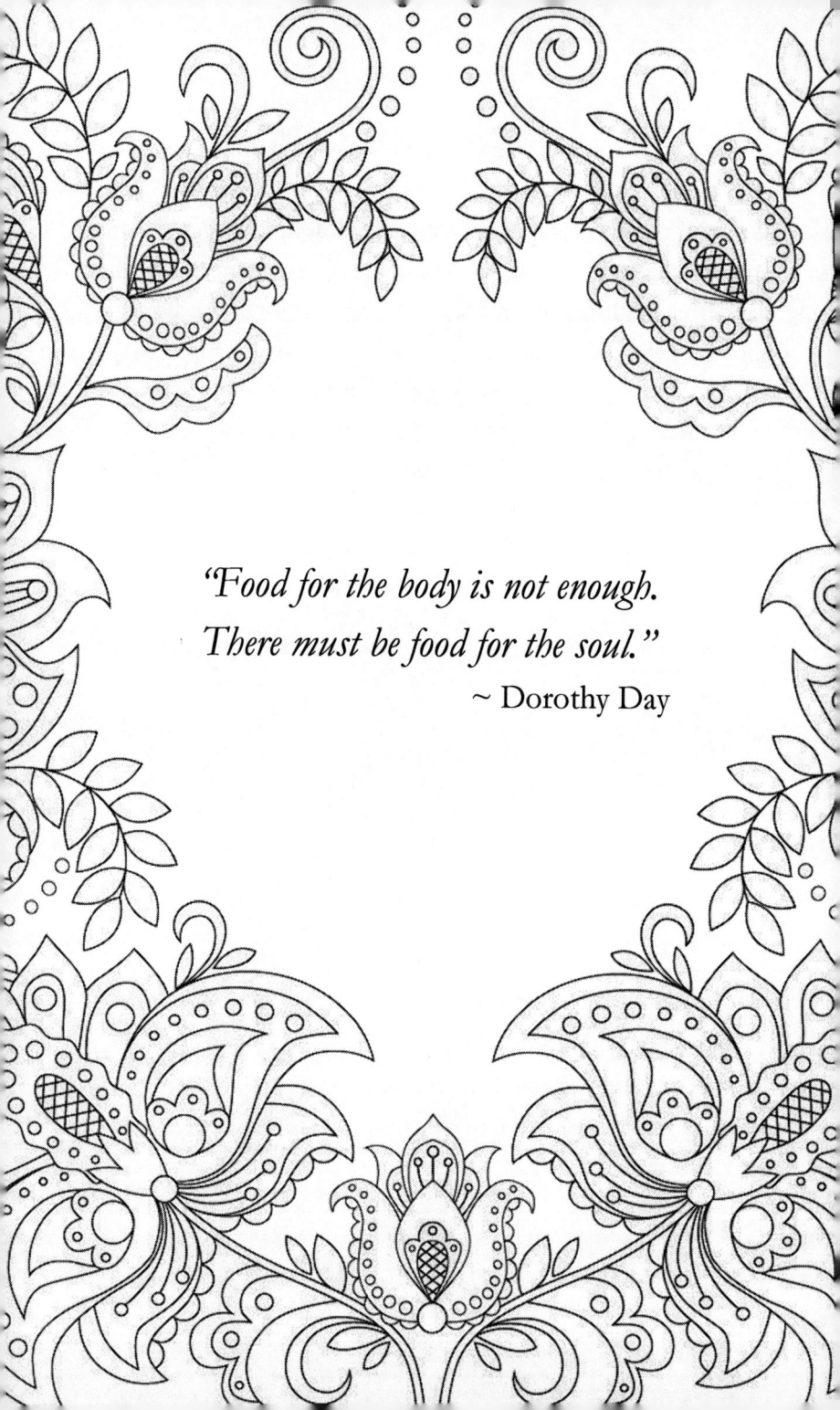

"Food for the body is not enough.
There must be food for the soul."

~ Dorothy Day

Chapter 8

Food

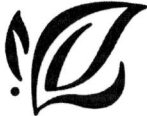

As I was writing this book, I was very surprised to find Food was my last Pillar. After all, it's a health book; food should at least be in the top three, right? Yes, food matters and is important, but what I have discovered from my personal journey, from training, from my clients, and from learning all I can about nutrition and health for the last 17 years, is that when we work on the other Pillars …

- Sleep

- Water

- Strong inner circle

- Stress management

- Movement

- Connection to something bigger

- Pockets of joy

… food has a way of working itself out. I'm not saying you don't have to educate yourself on what's nutritious, or be mindful of what you put into your body. I'm simply saying that the process unfolds in a natural way, if you allow it to. You will feel pulled—not pushed—to eat in a way that will serve you.

You'll naturally want to nourish your body and support it in a way that makes you feel alive and vibrant. Eating a meal turns into an expression of self-care. And when a healthy level of self-care kicks in, bad habits don't stand a chance. They just drop away.

Sometimes this happens all of a sudden, because you know what to do; other times you make a decision to take the time and get the education, support and accountability you need to make it happen. Either way, gone are the days of overthinking food and having it consume your life. You will no longer feel deprived over what you can't eat or how you can't get it done; instead, a deep appreciation and sweetness toward your body will ensue, and you will make the change. You will make it happen.

Food has always played a leading role in my life, and like most people, I had a love/love-not-so-much relationship with it. I started being more conscious of my body in high school, but it was during my college years that I really started watching what I ate and exercising intensively every day. My goal in college was to have a good body. From what I gathered, that meant being thin. I started paying attention to shows and ads on TV, I watched health talk shows, read the magazines, and unconsciously absorbed these images of what being beautiful and healthy looked like. I altered my diet and I bought into the standard nutritional advice of the time:

- Fat makes you *fat*.

- It's about counting calories.

- All calories are the same.

- It doesn't matter what you eat; if you want to lose weight, just consume fewer calories than you work off.

- Oh, and carbs are okay.

This advice didn't come out of thin air. It was based on information such as the USDA's food pyramid, which showcased breads, cereals, rice and pastas at the base of the pyramid, recommending up to 11 servings per day. Fats were placed right at the top, to be used sparingly. Those guidelines said nothing about sugar, refined carbs, processed and chemicalized foods, dyes, pesticides, hormones, ingredients you can't pronounce, "good" fats or "bad" fats. Just like many of you, I was interested in being healthy, and I trusted what the "experts" in health were saying. I trusted the doctors. I trusted the USDA guidelines and recommendations, and I trusted the health claims on boxes and packages of so-called food items.

It was not until I got sick in 1999 that I began questioning what I was actually eating, and reading labels, noticing how food affected my energy, sleep, weight, skin and mindset. My journey has led me to seek out the truth about nutrition, and how I could use food to heal my body. The beautiful thing about the world we live in is that when you seek out truth, there are already others that have paved a path; you just have to take the time to find them. And I did. There are so many people out there doing the work of rediscovering what it means to live a healthy lifestyle: traditionally trained medical doctors; integrative, functional and ayurvedic doctors; food activists; journalists, scientists; health coaches, and many, many more are out there doing great work. I have enrolled in their programs, read their books, articles and blogs, and have sifted through it all to find out what is true and what works for me, and I share it with my clients so they, too, can catch health.

Here's the thing: I am good with different practices when it comes to diet, as long as what you eat brings you vitality; there is no one right diet. Vegan or paleo or anything in between is fine—we are individuals, and we each have to figure out what works best for us. What I'm not good with is when we are manipulated into believing we are being healthy when we are clearly not.

I remember days in college when I would pass up homemade Indian lentils with healing, anti-inflammatory spices for a bowl of nonfat frozen yogurt with fat-free toppings. I also remember turning to a bowl of sugar-laden processed cereal with nonfat milk instead of a handful of nuts, because I thought nuts would make me fat. Back then, I didn't put as much emphasis on my own experience with food. I didn't ask the important questions like, *Do I feel nourished? Energized? Focused and fueled?* All I remember thinking about was, *Is that going to make me fat?* I didn't connect the extra weight I was carrying during those days to bad food; I attributed it to not working out enough. Remember, the messaging was that if you're not getting the results you wanted, you needed to burn more calories. So I did.

Our eating culture makes it very easy to push off a healthy lifestyle and/or just give up. Let me assure you right now, you can do it and it doesn't have to be complicated. Eating healthy is simple. Michael Pollan, journalist, food activist and five-time *New York Times* bestselling author synthesizes it in seven words: *Eat food, not too much, mostly plants.* The challenging part, due to the hijacking of our taste buds and hunger cues by a food industry that pushes heavily processed, overly sweetened snacks, will be getting rid of the junk.

All calories are not created equal. The quality of the food you eat matters and affects your immune, endocrine and digestive systems, affects your weight fluctuations, metabolism and ultimate wellness. Most people, even some doctors, still believe all calories are equal, and they think they're doing a good thing by counting calories. But this is a misleading belief. Unhealthy food leads to poor cell function, whereas healthy foods lead to healthy cell function. Bottom line: food has the power to bring health or harm to your body. What you eat and drink is literally bringing the outside world in, so choose wisely and intentionally. I have created several lists in the appendix of some of the healthiest, highest quality foods. Pick a few each week and incorporate them into your diet.

Having a healthy relationship with food means being relaxed around it and being confident that you will make healthful choices (at least 90% of the time) that are in line with your health and wellness goals. Eating is one of the most fundamental relationships we have with ourselves. Our food gives us the energy to live with vitality and wellness. The food we eat literally breaks down and becomes us.

How we eat is just as important as what we eat. Bringing mindfulness into your meals is a great way to connect to your own body. Mindful eating is a practice that not only leaves you feeling nourished and satisfied, but will take you to a space where you will naturally eat less and release extra weight. One of my favorite things to teach during my 21-Day Conscious

Cleanse is the art of mindful eating. Most of us are distracted while we eat our meals and snacks. We multi-task, even while eating, by watching TV or playing on our devices. We eat on the go in our cars, or while we're running from one errand to the next. After I had children, my eating patterns changed because of time constraints. I started eating faster and less mindfully. This is a bad combination because you miss-out on the eating experience and you end up eating more. It's important for our health and well-being to sit down at least once a day and enjoy our meal. Whether you're by yourself or with people, take the time to relax during your meals. Start with just one meal a day for the next three weeks and notice how your relationship with food shifts. I refer to mindful eating as a "yoga meal." Yoga is a practice of inviting in presence, and that is exactly what I want to do while I eat. Bringing the moment in while you eat will connect you to the natural intelligence of the body. Incorporating at least one yoga meal will help you slow down, digest and connect—give it a go.

Yoga Meal Guidelines:

- For this meal remain seated at the table (no car, no TV, no reading, no distractions).

- Pause before you start. Take three deep breaths (awaken your senses and invoke a sense of gratitude toward what you are about to receive).

- Every bite you take should be fully chewed before you swallow; put the fork down while you chew. Salivary amylase is an enzyme located in the mouth that is released when you chew. This is the beginning of the digestion process.

- Wait till the food is fully digested before your next meal or snack. Take some time to experience real hunger. Not eating because you're bored, angry, stressed or even happy. Eat only when you are hungry.

- Make breakfast a medium-sized meal. Lunch should be your largest, as digestive juices are the strongest then, leaving dinner to be your smallest.

- Do what the Okinawans do—*hara hachi bu*, which means eat until you are 80% full.

- Eat 2–3 high protein/good fat and fiber snacks.

Eating this way will increase your energy. Digesting food takes an enormous amount of energy, and as we slow things down, we help the digestive process along. Eating this way also cuts down on how much we eat, because by slowing down, we reduce the delay between the quantity of food consumed and the brain registering that we are full. Mindful eaters tend not to overeat. They taste, savor and enjoy every bite. Even when I eat with people, I take in my food with the same concepts. Remember: *hara hachi bu*.

Earlier I mentioned making the right food choices 90% of the time. Let's talk about that last 10% for a moment. When you do choose to eat a decadent dessert or a favorite not-so healthy snack or meal, make sure you make the decision *consciously*. I tell my clients all the time, if you desire a not-so healthy dessert or meal, it's okay. Just decide, sit your butt down, and mindfully make out with it. Be completely there, you will connect and feel satiated sooner. The magic of bringing the moment into your daily life as much as possible is that your body's natural intelligence takes over. With this practice, you will never leave a table stuffed, because you will know when to say when.

When most of us think of losing weight or getting healthier, we tend to focus on what we have to give-up and sacrifice. We come to it from a place of deprivation and lack. The foods we have to give up, the joy those foods give us, we might feel our social life will suffer and that life will become boring and just not as fun.

I say this with love, but that's a load of crap.

I invite you to shift that mindset. For human beings to make lasting changes, we must feel connected to the change. We must feel invested, and that we are a part of a greater outcome. This is something I do with my Health Coaching Clients, and I want to share it with you. I get them excited about changing. Before we even go into making changes with what they eat, I ask them several questions to help facilitate this mindset shift. I start by telling them not to be concerned about the how(s) right now, and just to imagine what their life would be like if they had this weight thing handled.

Ask Yourself …

- How would you be different in the world if you lost the extra weight?

- How would it feel if living a healthy lifestyle was a priority, and you did it with ease and joy?

- What would you do with all this newfound energy and sense of wellness?

- Why is it so important to you in this stage of your life?

- Who will be affected?

- What's stopping you?

- Why is it important for you to change right now?

- If you don't change, what will your life be like in one year? Three years? Ten years?

My job as an Integrative Health Coach is to create urgency around making the changes. I want people to get excited about their lives and take charge. Most people never take the time to step back and take a look at where their lives are going, they just put it on auto-pilot and hope for the best. Change does not happen by doing the same old thing. If we truly desire a different result, we must do something different.

This can be a challenge, with all the contradictory theories and diets out there on what's good for you and what's not. Every week there seems to be a new study or article that debunks the previous week's study. It's constantly changing and it is confusing, but I think we are making it more complicated than it has to be. Let's just start with what we know. We don't have to go to extremes and cut out entire food groups, but we do know there are certain foods most experts can agree are not good for us. Let's start there.

Some examples: sugar in all its forms (I have provided a list of all its aliases in the appendix); processed and refined flours; trans fats (aka hydrogenated or partially hydrogenated);

vegetable and seed oils like soybean, canola, sunflower, safflower, corn, peanut and cottonseed oils; artificial sweeteners; preservatives; artificial colors; and additives like MSG—staying away from just these items will eliminate foods with a long shelf life. (This is not going to sound sexy, but the food we eat should be capable of rotting. It should go bad. We want to consume live food, not dead, engineered food-like junk.)

For good health and vitality, we require fresh, nutrient-dense, whole foods. Sounds simple, right?

Simple, maybe—but not easy. Almost everyone I know is on a diet, or trying to get healthy. It's been a challenge, and requires a more holistic approach. Knowing what real food is and isn't, knowing how our bodies react and get addicted to these overly processed foods, and knowing that we can start where we are and make changes, will empower us to *want* to make better choices.

I don't put you on a strict eating plan, I don't have you measure food or count calories; I just invite you to add in more nutrient-dense, whole foods. Getting the best food you can afford is where I would start.

Revamping what and how you eat can feel overwhelming, so don't hesitate because you think you can't do it all perfectly. Just start. One of the core concepts that I fell in love with during my nutrition training at Integrative Nutrition was the concept of "crowding out," which means putting more of your attention on adding the good, healthy stuff to your diet, as opposed to spending your attention on avoiding the unhealthy ones. The idea is that, when you start eating more of the good stuff, your palate and preferences begin to shift, and eventually all the junky foods get crowded out. This happens with less deprivation and struggle. So instead of thinking lack or giving up, just get in there and start exploring by bringing in some new delicious, healthful foods. Again, I'll refer you to the Appendix for more details and suggestions.

I have to admit, writing this chapter has been challenging for me. I struggled with narrowing down what information would be most helpful for you on your health journey. I think there is already enough confusion and frustration around food. My intention for this chapter was to keep it very simple and give you a good framework, and then share all the best foods I have discovered from my trainings, readings and experience. As mentioned above, the concept of crowding out is what I invite you to focus on. The idea is to add in the highest quality of nutrient-dense whole foods you can afford, and allow the junk to fall away. Your job is to see how your body responds. Everyone's body is different, and some people can tolerate higher amounts of certain foods than others.

I invite you to add in the good stuff and let your body take care of the rest. Your body knows what to do with real food. It was masterfully designed that way. Give it a chance—all you have to do is create the environment for true healing and health to happen.

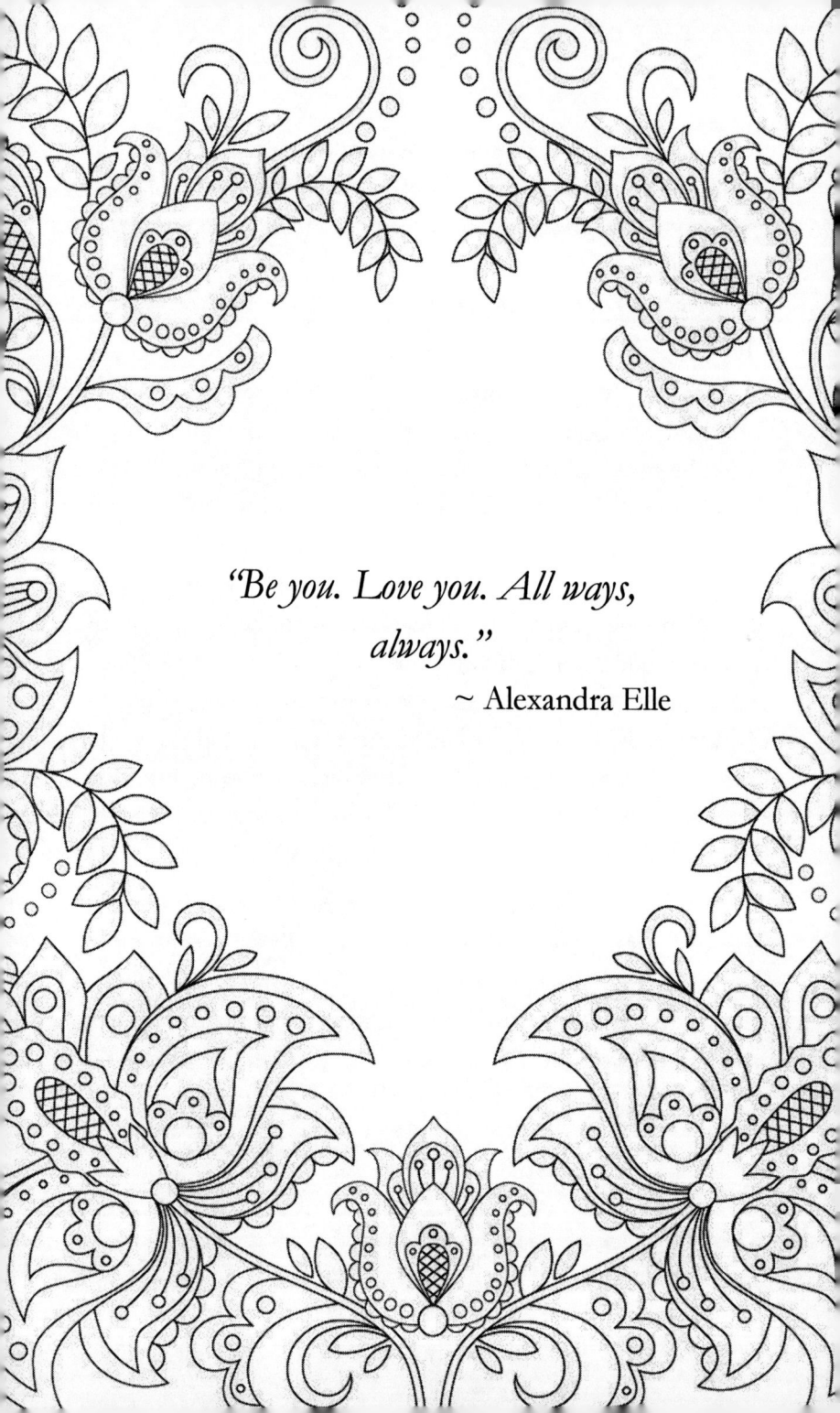

"Be you. Love you. All ways, always."

~ Alexandra Elle

Chapter 9

Self-Love—Putting It All Together

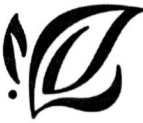

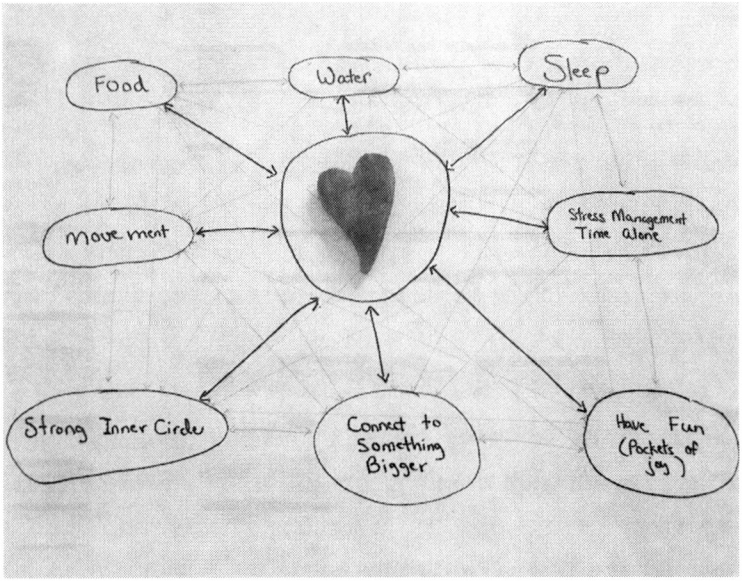

When I decided to write this book, one of the first things I did was map it out on a board. Fine-tuning the Pillars, and without much thought, what I discovered was that they all came from the same place. The road to Health and Wholeness is building these Eight Pillars, but the center is connected to self-love. Please, don't wait until you have lost the weight or gotten healthy before you treat yourself well. Exquisite kindness toward yourself, forgiveness and love is the fuel that will spark true wellness. Come from a place of love, compassion and okay-ness about your body and how it got here. Give yourself the gift of loving and appreciating your body now, as is, and watch how change happens. Your change will come from a different energy. Carl Rogers, an American psychologist (1902-1987), who is considered one of the founding fathers of psychotherapy research, names this very thing The Curious Paradox: *"The curious paradox is that when I accept myself just as I am, then I change."*

Most of us spend too much energy on what's not working and how we're not enough. Just the idea of accepting who we are right now, with all our imperfections, has the power to shift our focus. Practice acceptance and self-love every day, as you are, and let go of anything else. Real change happens when we feel a sense of clarity, presence and hope.

If you're not at a place of giving yourself this kind of acceptance or self-love, I would recommend doing mirror work. Louise Hay not only taught me about affirmations, but also about mirror work. This is a simple activity you can do to wake up and connect with that loving place within you. This space is always there, all we have to do is bring it out. Give it a go.

- Make sure you will not be disturbed.

- Either get a hand mirror or stand/sit in front of a mirror.

- Look at your face. Look into your eyes.

- Really look at yourself without judgment or critique. Look deep into your eyes, moving from one to the other.

- Breathe. Be with yourself.

- The first time you do this, you might feel a little weird or uncertain if you're doing it right. As long as you're looking at yourself without judgment, you're good.

- Say out loud, "I love you." Pause.

- Say it again, "I love you."

- Don't disengage. Keep your eye contact. "I love you."

- Notice what comes up and just be with it.

The first time I did this, I sobbed. I felt so much compassion for the reflection I witnessed. I felt love for this scared girl I witnessed. I didn't look away, I stayed with her and my own reflection. This activity opened my heart and gave me strength. I have done this exercise so many times since, but that initial spark has never left me, that compassion and care for myself has only grown. I believe in the deepest part of me that when you truly see yourself without judgment and feel love for all of you (even the broken parts) you will heal. And as you heal, you will naturally take care of yourself.

All Eight Pillars are important for lasting health and wholeness. They create a solid foundation, so no matter what's going on in your life or whatever phase you are in, you will be able to take care of you. There is no exact order in how to start, it depends where you are and what in your life needs more attention and love. As I mentioned earlier, if you're feeling completely overwhelmed, I would recommend water and sleep. Pick one or two Pillars and commit to incorporating them into your life every day. Remember, it's the small things we do every day that create massive changes. Once you get it humming along in your daily life, then add in something else. Also, don't worry if it's not a linear progression. If you get off track or feel overwhelmed, pull back and return to what feels doable. It's always going to be about progress and never about attaining perfection. You might have heard the saying, *perfection is the enemy of the good.* Too often, striving for perfection is the reason we give up and never reach our goals, desires or even dreams.

Just start.

- You will eat whole, nutrient-dense foods.

- Drink plenty of water.

- Get quality sleep.

- Movement will be a priority.

- Stress will be managed.

- You will deepen your inner circle.

- You will connect to something bigger.

- And, lastly you will have fun. Pockets of joy will be infused into your day and into your life.

All these things will come once you rediscover that place in your heart. Self-love leads to self-care, and self-care naturally brings health. No more chasing; all you have to do is love yourself, live consciously and catch it.

I hope this book serves you and sheds light on ideas or simple things you can do, starting right now, to bring you more health, happiness, and love. You deserve it, and remember you *were* never and *will* never be broken. You are a masterpiece.

The only real question left is, are *you* ready?

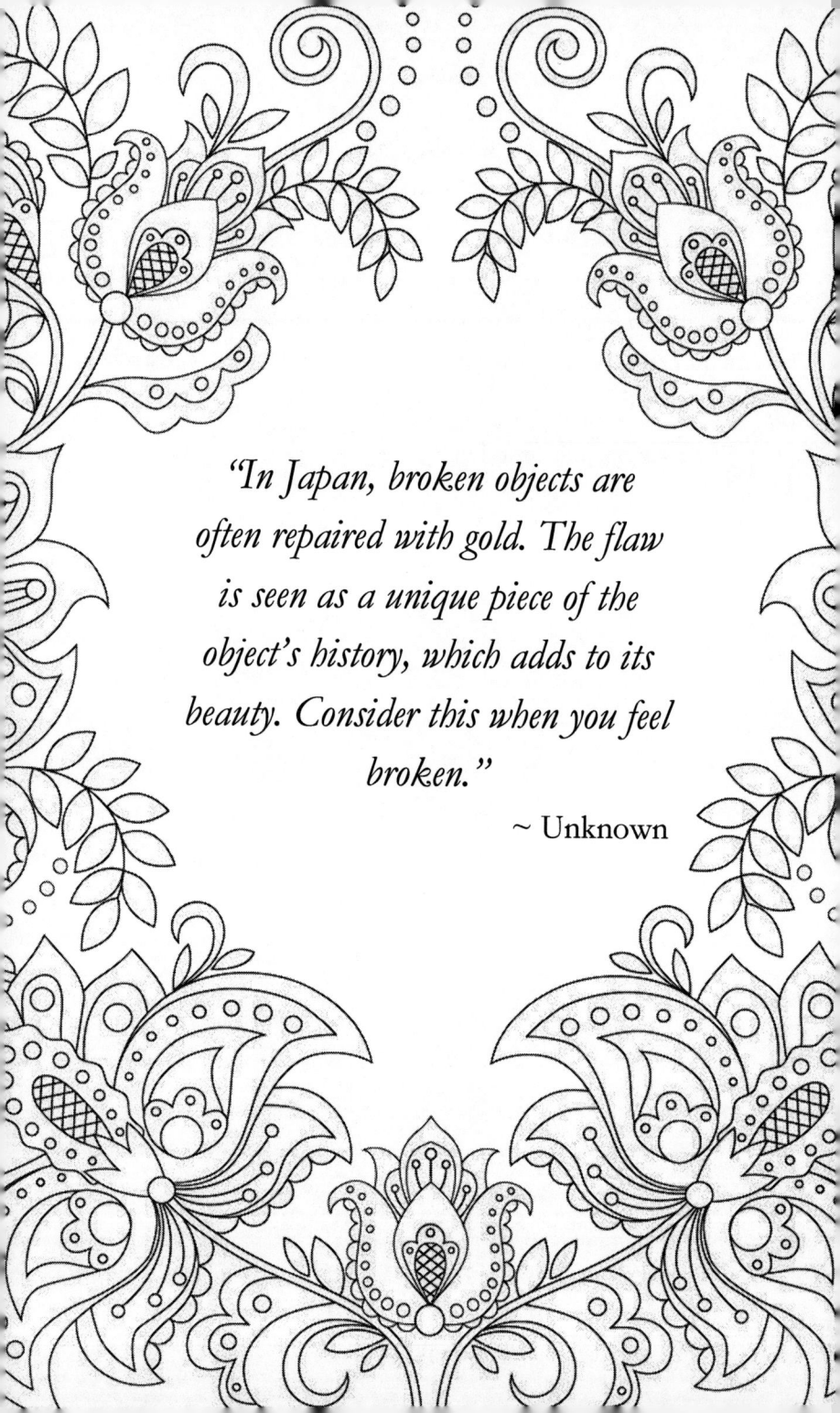

"In Japan, broken objects are often repaired with gold. The flaw is seen as a unique piece of the object's history, which adds to its beauty. Consider this when you feel broken."

~ Unknown

Private Health Coaching Special Offer

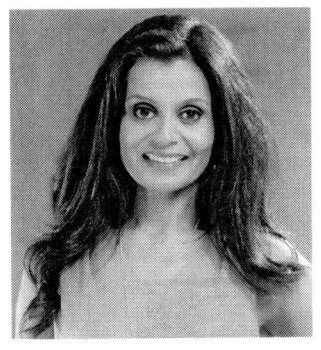

I hope the words on these pages have served you and have given you a few things to think about … and maybe even implement right away. Remember, taking action gets this whole thing going, so just start!

Rita Hari is an Integrative Health Coach, yoga teacher and author. Her clients have had sustainable success because she comes from a place of mindfulness and self-care. She teaches them how to:

- Reconnect and rediscover their own healing properties.

- Identify their limiting thoughts, beliefs and old patterns—places of "stuckness."

- Get super clear on what they want.

- Be accountable in taking daily actions to reach their desired goals.

- Make better quality choices of food and other lifestyle habits. She calls these choices "upgrades."

This personalized road map will bring health, increased energy, weight loss, glowing skin and just feeling good. This helps clients clear the pathway so they can *Live Consciously, Catch Health* … and maybe even chase their dreams. It's all possible with the right support.

If you found the book helpful and want to take the next step, please, go to my website at www.ritahariwellness.com and sign-up for my program (four, eight or twelve 1-hour sessions). Invest in your health. It is your most vital asset. Let me know you read my book and get a special discount worth $75-150, depending on the program you purchase.

Thank you again, I look forward to one day meeting you on your health journey. Wishing you health and wholeness … always.

xoxo,

Rita Hari

Appendix: Notes on What to Eat (and What Not to)

Following are lists of healthy foods that you can use to "crowd out" the not-so-good. Below those are some foods that are worth avoiding.

Healthy Foods

Low-Glycemic Fruits: The natural sugar in fruits isn't terrible, but it's still worth keeping an eye on. Following is a list of low-glycemic fruits that won't spike your sugar levels.

- All berries.
- Cherries.
- Grapefruit.
- Peaches.
- Apricots.
- Apples.
- Oranges.
- Pomegranate seeds.
- Pears.
- Kiwi.
- Grapes.
- Lemons/Limes.

Vegetables: Go crazy! Really, eat as much as you want, as long as it's not deep-fried in oil or sugar-coated!

- Artichokes.

- Asparagus.

- Avocados (I know, not a vegetable—just eat them)

- Bamboo shoots.

- Bean sprouts.

- Beets.

- Bell peppers (all colors).

- Broccoli.

- Broccoli rabe.

- Brussels sprouts.

- Cabbage (green, bok choy, Chinese).

- Carrots.

- Cauliflower.

- Celery.

- Cucumbers.

- Daikon.

- Eggplant.

- Fennel.

- Garlic.

- Ginger.

- Green beans.

- Greens (collard, kale, Swiss chard, mustard, turnip).

- Heart of palm.

- Jalapenos.

- Jicama.

- Leeks.

- Mushrooms (all types).

- Okra.

- Onions.

- Parsley.

- Parsnips.

- Radishes.

- Rutabaga.

- Salad greens (chicory, endive, escarole, lettuce, romaine, spinach, arugula, radicchio, watercress, red and green leaf lettuce).

- Seaweeds.

- Squash (spaghetti).

- Sweet potatoes.

- Tomatoes.

- Water chestnuts.

- Zucchini.

Fresh Herbs:

- Basil.

- Chives.

- Cilantro.

- Dill.

- Lemongrass.

- Mint.

- Oregano.

- Tarragon.

- Parsley.

- Sage.

- Rosemary.

- Thyme.

Healthy Fats (think Omega 3's):

- Organic cold-pressed extra virgin olive oil.

- Ghee (purified butter).

- Organic grass-fed butter.

- Organic unrefined coconut oil.
- Avocado oil.
- Flaxseed and hempseed oil.
- Avocados.

Beans and Legumes (Vegetarian Protein):

- Garbanzo beans.
- All lentils.
- Black and pinto beans.
- Lima beans.
- Kidney beans.
- White beans (cannellini, navy, great north).

Nuts, Seeds and Nut Butters (choose raw):

- Almonds, cashews, walnuts, pine nuts, pecans, macadamias.
- Chia, hemp, pumpkin, sunflower, flax, sesame.
- Almond and Cashew butter.
- Tahini.

Spices and Dried Herbs (Choose organic when you can):

- All the fresh herbs come in dry form, too.
- Cumin, turmeric, paprika, red pepper flakes, garlic powder, sea salt, curry, cayenne, cinnamon.

Dairy:

- I limit dairy consumption. If I use cow's milk for Indian chai or certain recipes that call for milk, I only use organic, pasture-raised whole milk (never low or non-fat).

- Kefir (full fat).

- Greek yogurt (full fat, plain—add your own berries).

- Unsweetened almond, coconut or hemp milk.

- Cheese—again I limit cheese intake. When I do eat it, it's high quality + small quantity. (Grass-fed sharp cheddar is my favorite.)

- Grass-fed butter.

Grains, Breads and my favorite noodles (Cut back on the gluten, and small quantities):

- Ezekiel bread.

- Whole-kernel rye bread.

- Steel-cut oats.

- Quinoa.

- Brown or wild rice.

- Soba noodles (made from buckwheat).

Seafood (low mercury, wild, fresh or canned fish):

- Salmon.

- Sardines.

- Herring.

- Mackerel.

- Black cod (sablefish).

- Shrimp.

- Crab.

- Mussels.

- Scallops.

Meat and Eggs

- Know where your meat comes from; ideally, organic, pasture-raised, grass-fed animals. You can go a step further and buy from small farms where the animals are treated well and are fed a proper diet.

- Eat meat in moderation, a couple of times a week. The size of your palm is a good portion (4–6 ounces).

- Eat eggs that come from chickens that eat grass and play outside. Cage-free, free-range or organic is not good enough—eat *pasture-raised* eggs. These eggs taste better, are healthier, and the chickens are humanely treated. It's a win-win.

Drinks:

- Water with lemon.

- I do drink 1-2 cups of organic coffee per day. If drinking coffee does not agree with you or keeps you from a good night's sleep (see Chapter 3), then don't drink it.

- Herbal or green teas.

- Wine (red or white), just one glass 3–4 times a week.

- Green smoothies/juices.

Vinegars/Condiments:

- Bragg's Organic Apple Cider.

- White and red wine.

- Balsamic.

- Tamari (gluten-free soy sauce).

- Nutritional yeast.

- Hot sauce (no sugar).

- Dijon mustard.

Sweets and Sweeteners (small amounts):

- Raw, organic honey.

- 100% pure maple syrup.

- Cacao nibs/powder.

- Goji berries.

- Unsweetened dried cherries.

- Dark Chocolate (80% cacao).

Not-so-Healthy Foods

Stay Away From or Limit the Amount of:

- Pesticides, antibiotics or hormones, additives, preservatives, dyes, MSG, artificial sweeteners and GMO's.

- Hydrogenated (trans fat) oils and refined vegetable and seed oils, which include corn, soy, canola, sunflower and safflower.

- Processed carbohydrates (you know, the snacks that fill up the grocery store aisles with long ingredient lists, long shelf life, and processed, refined flours and sugars).

- Anything that is not real food.

- Sugar, no matter what fancy name they call it, added in any food or drinks.

Sugar Aliases

Agave nectar	Crystalized fructose	Lactose
Agave syrup	Date sugar	Malt
Barley malt	Dextran	Maltodextrin
Beet sugar	Dextrose	Maltose
Brown rice syrup	Diastatic malt	Maple syrup
Brown sugar	Evaporated cane juice	Molasses
Buttered syrup	Fructose	Raw sugar
Cane sugar	Fruit juice	Refiner's syrup
Cane juice	Fruit juice concentrate	Soghum syrup
Cane juice crystals	Glucose	Sucanat
Carob syrup	Glucose solids	Sucrose
Confectioner's sugar	Golden sugar	Sugar
Corn syrup	Golden syrup	Turbindo sugar
High fructose corn syrup	Grape sugar	Yellow sugar
Corn sugar	Grape juice concentrate	
Corn sweetener	Honey	
Corn syrup solids	Invert sugar	

When you cut out or drastically reduce sugar, you will find yourself automatically eating less gluten. Gluten is a protein found in most breads, cereals, and pastas. Getting the bready stuff out is a good habit, and will have you feeling lighter and cleaner in no time. This is another common habit around lean people with healthy lifestyles, they limit their bread, and if they do partake, they eat the kind that goes hard within a day or two.

Buying Organic

If you're new to the whole organic trend, no worries. It's a lot to take in, and it can get expensive. Fortunately, because more and more American consumers are voting (with their pocketbooks) for produce with less pesticide, whole organic sections have appeared in regular grocery stores, making organic foods more accessible.

For more options, check out the resources below:

- Local Harvest, a guide to finding locally raised/grown food near you: www.localharvest.org.

- A free app to find farmers markets near you: www.farmstandapp.com.

- Environmental Working Group, a not-for-profit group that educates consumers about pesticides and other environmental issues: www.ewg.org.

As I mentioned in Chapter 8, Food, if you can't afford to go all-organic immediately, you can at least start replacing some of the worst pesticide offenders (the "dirty dozen") with their organic equivalents and continuing to buy non-organic versions of the "clean fifteen," which are very low in pesticides.

Dirty Dozen	Clean Fifteen
1. Strawberries.	1. Avocados.
2. Apples.	2. Corn.
3. Nectarines.	3. Pineapples.
4. Peaches.	4. Cabbage.
5. Celery.	5. Sweet peas(Frozen).
6. Grapes.	6. Onions.
7. Cherries.	7. Asparagus.
8. Spinach.	8. Mangoes.
9. Tomatoes.	9. Papayas.
10. Bell peppers.	10. Kiwi.
11. Cherry tomatoes.	11. Eggplant.
12. Cucumbers.	12. Honeydew Melon.
	13. Grapefruit.
	14. Cantaloupe.
	15. Cauliflower.

CPSIA information can be obtained
at www.ICGtesting.com
Printed in the USA
FFOW04n1005160217
32530FF